The Anti-Estrogenic Diet

The Anti-Estrogenic Diet

How Estrogenic Foods and Chemicals Are Making You Fat and Sick

Ori Hofmekler

author of *The Warrior Diet*

with Rick Osborn

North Atlantic Books
Berkeley, California

Published by North Atlantic Books
P.O. Box 12327   Cover and book design by Brad Greene
Berkeley, California 94712   Printed in the United States of America

The Anti-Estrogenic Diet: How Estrogenic Foods and Chemicals Are Making You Fat and Sick is sponsored by the Society for the Study of Native Arts and Sciences, a non-profit educational corporation whose goals are to develop an educational and cross-cultural perspective linking various scientific, social, and artistic fields; to nurture a holistic view of arts, sciences, humanities, and healing; and to publish and distribute literature on the relationship of mind, body, and nature.

MEDICAL DISCLAIMER: The following information is intended for general information purposes only. Individuals should always see their health care provider before administering any suggestions made in this book. Any application of the material set forth in the following pages is at the reader's discretion and is his or her sole responsibility.

North Atlantic Books' publications are available through most bookstores. For further information, call 800-337-2665 or visit our website at www.northatlanticbooks.com.

Substantial discounts on bulk quantities are available to corporations, professional associations, and other organizations. For details and discount information, contact our special sales department.

Library of Congress Cataloging-in-Publication Data

Hofmekler, Ori, 1952–
    The anti-estrogenic diet : how estrogenic foods and chemicals are making you fat and sick / by Ori Hofmekler.
        p. cm.
    Includes bibliographical references.
    ISBN-13: 978-1-55643-684-0
    ISBN-10: 1-55643-684-X
    1. Anti-estrogenic diet. 2. Estrogen—Toxicology. 3. Food—Estrogen content. I. Title.
RM231.2.H64 2007
615.9'02—dc22
                                                                2006103186
                                                                CIP

1 2 3 4 5 6 7 8 9 VERSA 14 13 12 11 10 09 08 07

In loving memory of my mom,
Rina

Acknowledgments

I'd like to thank my family and friends who encouraged me to write this book. I'd also like to thank Erich Bumgardner for his generous support and wise advice. Rick Osborn made important contributions in the editing and designing of the book. I'd like to thank Gary Choma for his hard work, help, and diligence on this project. Special thanks to my literary agent Bill Stranger for his support and professional advice.

I'd also like to express my gratitude to all Warrior Diet certified trainers and coaches, and in particular, Barry Bragg and Barry Seneri, who were passionately dedicated to helping gather testimonials for the program and address commonly asked questions.

Last, but not least, I thank my wife Natasha for being my biggest supporter in times when I really needed someone to watch my back.

Table of Contents

A Note from the Author

I've been following a diet that breaks all conventional rules. I eat as much as I want. I eat only food that I like. I also enjoy overeating and snacking while relaxing in front of TV late at night. While most people around me are struggling not to gain weight, I find it difficult to keep my weight from dropping. I can't even remember the last time I had to visit a doctor.

This may seem too good to be true, but it isn't. Here is why. The diet that I practice incorporates certain nutritional elements that are surprisingly missing in most other diets. I believe that these very elements are what keep me lean and healthy. As you'll soon realize, without these nutritional elements, any diet would be doomed to failure.

The purpose of this book is to guide you on how to incorporate these critical nutritional elements into your daily routine. These elements are critical because they can help provide you with the means to defend your life.

Whether you are aware of it or not, you are constantly exposed to an assault of chemicals known for causing hormonal imbalance, disorders, and death—chemicals that are found in the air you breathe, products you use, lotions you put on your skin, food you eat, and water you drink.

These chemicals act in your body like the female hormone estrogen, causing estrogen disorders in women, feminization and sterilization of men, and some of the deadliest cancers in humankind. To make matters worse, estrogenic chemicals exist in both synthetic and natural forms. The synthetic forms, called xenoestrogens, are industrial derivatives, whereas the natural forms, called phytoestrogens, naturally occur in certain foods, herbs, and extracts. The double whammy of being exposed to both synthetic and natural estrogens has an overwhelming effect on the body.

How can we defend ourselves when it's almost impossible to avoid these estrogenic substances? This is not a simple question to answer.

We are currently facing a major ecological problem. These very chemicals, already known for causing the near extinction of various living species today, are currently threatening our own survival. Yet, this problem is not addressed by any current dietary program. There are many articles and studies that provide much information about the problem but very little about the solution.

The Anti-Estrogenic Diet is about solutions. It incorporates nutritional elements that help counterbalance excess of estrogens. It goes head-to-head against common nutritional concepts, but presents an effective program based on science, epidemiology, and life experience.

Statistically, most diets today fail in the long run. Obviously, something must be wrong with those diets. This book explains why diets fail and exposes dietary myths and fallacies. You will learn how wrong your food choices can be in spite of all good intentions. For that matter, you will realize how some of the most popular health-food items today may actually cause weight gain and disorders, whereas some of the foods that you may have been led to believe are fattening can, in fact, help you become lean and healthy.

The following chapters provide you with practical advice that will very likely appeal to your personal needs, lifestyle, and even ethnic background. Most frequent questions are addressed in the Q & A chapter towards the end of the book.

You can start practicing the program immediately. Begin with the diet's Jump-Start, Week 1, and you may be able to notice some initial results before even finishing the book. Over time, you may be able to improve the way you look and the way you feel. You may also notice a thinning-down effect in areas that previously resisted fat burning, such as around the belly. By improving your metabolic state, you may be able to reverse existing health conditions. And finally, you'll be able to enjoy eating the foods that you like without the typical side effects or guilt.

Like all humans, you carry within you awesome survival mechanisms. All you need is the knowledge to trigger them. Once triggered, they will provide you with all the energy and health that you need to better survive. Take advantage of your innate power. Nourish yourself properly, live better, and live longer.

—Ori Hofmekler

Introduction

Excess Estrogen in the Environment and Food

There is too much estrogen in the world today. Never before has the human body been exposed to such an overwhelming amount of estrogenic substances. Most of our conventional food is estrogenic. Our meat and dairy are loaded with hormones and our vegetables and fruits are treated with pesticides, all of which virtually mimic estrogen activity in our bodies. Our animal food is mostly female. The male animal that we eat is either castrated (capon) or treated with estrogen to tenderize the meat. We have never adapted to such a surplus of estrogen in our food and environment, nor have our genes been programmed for such estrogen dominance.

Over-Feminization of the World

As a consequence of this imbalance, there is a process of over-feminization that is being noted around the world. Certain species of marine life are becoming sterile and virtually extinct due to petroleum contamination, plasticizers, and other estrogenic chemicals in the oceans, rivers, and lakes. Men, women, and children today are notably getting fatter and heavier due to the effects of excess estrogen. The rates of estrogen-related disorders and cancer in both sexes have reached almost epidemic proportions.

The Anti-Estrogenic Diet

The world today has lost its ecological balance. It is becoming overly feminized by these estrogenic chemicals and estrogenic foods, and there isn't enough anti-estrogenic food in our diet. Ironically, many health-food and weight-loss products, including protein bars and shakes, are made with soy protein and petroleum-based chemical additives that promote estrogen.

Something must be done to fight this excess of estrogen. That something requires the incorporation of anti-estrogenic foods and nutrients. It also requires a virtual elimination of estrogen-promoting food and chemicals. The term "nutrition" must be redefined to declare war against excess estrogen. This new concept is literally the core of the Anti-Estrogenic Diet.

Such a dietary approach may cause controversy and initial resistance. Regardless, all of us—men and women alike—need to follow an anti-estrogenic diet today in order to better survive. We require food and nutrients that can help support our hormonal integrity—nutrition that can help counter the already existing dominance of estrogen. We need food that makes us leaner, stronger, and healthier, food that fits our genes—food that is too often deficient in our diets.

In the pages that follow, you'll find information on healthy living, recipes for healthy eating, and reports of the hows and whys of how the excess of estrogen affects us. For those who'd like more technical information, we've provided many references. Where a reference is not indicated, you should consult the very thorough survey article by I. C. Munro and colleagues (2003) listed in the reference section.

Introduction

As bold as it may seem to be, the Anti-Estrogenic Diet is the only effective way to provide the body with a nutritional means to fight excess estrogen.

Chapter 1

Is Our Very Survival Being Threatened by Estrogenic Chemicals?

Estrogenic chemicals produced industrially, also known as xeno-estrogens, are a large, diverse group of chemical compounds that can mimic estrogen and interfere with the body's hormonal activities. Evidence is accumulating that xenoestrogens can disrupt sexual development and reproductive functions of various living species. Some of these chemicals that have penetrated our rivers and ponds—such as plasticizers and petroleum compounds—have been found to cause severe damaging effects on wildlife marine species. Examples of such effects include a decline in the sperm quality of fish, interference with the sexual development of alligators and turtles, and the feminization of male frogs. Researchers found recently that about 40% of male bass in the Potomac River (Washington DC) were producing eggs. Other feminization signs of male fish were found in the Colorado River in white sucker fish. Researchers at the University of California, Berkeley, found that a commonly used weed killer, atrazine, caused severe feminization and sterilization of frogs. Researchers believe that chronic exposure to estrogenic chemicals may lead to the virtual extinction of some wildlife species.

● ● ● **Unfortunately, the same chemicals known for causing feminization, sterilization, and the near extinction of various living species today are also found in some of the most common things—the food we eat and the water we drink.**

Unfortunately, the same chemicals known for causing feminization, sterilization, and the near extinction of various living species are also found in some of the most common things—the food we eat and the water we drink.

According to Turner, et al., environmental estrogens have been shown to inhibit human sperm production. Xenoestrogens are also suspected of causing breast cancer cells and vaginal epithelial cells proliferation (Krishnan et al.; Long et al.).

Xenoestrogens, Chemical Castration, and Cancer

There is evidence that estrogenic chemicals cause devastating effects on male potency and capacity to reproduce. Exposure of lab species and wildlife to estrogenic chemicals was found to cause abnormalities in the reproductive tract. Xenoestrogens have shown the ability to bind to estrogen receptors in different glands in both animals and humans, including the gonads, hypothalamus, and pituitary, thereby interrupting their normal functions. For that matter, xenoestrogens were found to adversely affect testicular gene expression, and also to cause changes in the hypothalamic-pituitary axis in the brain, which is responsible for the healthy regulation of estrogen.

Estrogen is not a single hormone, but rather a group of steroid hormones and their bioactive metabolites. Unlike with other steroid hormones, estrogen receptors are found both in the nucleus and the plasma membrane of cells. That may explain why xenoestrogens have such a high capacity for mimicking estrogen.

For example, the chemical BSA (conjugated estradiol) is a large compound that is unable to gain entry into the cytosol. Nonetheless, it can still bind to estrogen receptors in the plasma membrane and induce an estrogenic effect. This chemical, also known as synthetic estrogen, was found to cause decreased testicular androgen production in men. BSA is routinely used in commercially raised livestock to fatten the animals to increase profitability. BSA is also commonly found in the meat we eat (commercial beef, chicken, and pork).

Xenoestrogens have shown the ability to induce aromatase activity. Aromatase is the enzyme responsible for synthesis of estrogen from the androgens—male hormones. Studies showed that over-expression of the aromatase gene and enhanced estradiol production in mice induced spermatogenesis arrest and decreased serum testosterone levels. Over time, estrogenic chemicals caused progressive degeneration of testicular tissues and sexual behavioral problems in rodents.

● ● ● **Elevated blood estrogen levels are known to increase the risk of testicular cancer in men.**

The harmful effects of xenoestrogens are also evident in humans. A recent study involving a large cohort of men concluded that exposure to the chemical diethylstilbestrol (DES) caused testicular cancer and malformation of the genitals. DES is one out of several estrogenic chemicals used as a pharmaceutical agent. Researchers believe that the current increased incidence of testicular cancer in men is most likely due to fetal exposure to estrogenic chemicals, which interfere with the ability of gonadal steroids to support normal tissue differentiation in utero. Elevated blood-estrogen levels are known to increase the risk of testicular cancer in men.

Recent studies at the University of Texas provided evidence that explains the distinct abilities of xenoestrogens to disrupt reproductive functions even at low concentrations. Researchers tested various xenoestrogens including the phytoestrogen cumestriol (found in soy), organochlorine pesticides and their metabolites (endosulfan, dieldrin, and DDE), and detergent byproducts of plastic manufacturing (p-nonylphenol and bisphenol A). The result showed that these xenoestrogens produced rapid estrogen receptor activation (3–30 minutes after application). Furthermore, the same xenoestrogens were also found to be capable of binding and activating estrogen receptors in the pituitary tumor cell line, which expresses high levels of membrane receptors for estrogen.

The pharmaceutical industry argues that xenoestrogens are generally much weaker than the naturally occurring hormone estrogen and therefore unable to compete and induce estrogenic activity. However, there is enough evidence to show that xenoestrogens can bind to estrogen receptors and produce rapid changes in signaling effects, similar to estradiol, the estrogen produced in the ovaries (Chen et al. 1999; Levin et al. 1999; Norfleet et al. 1999; Pappas et al. 1994).

Xenoestrogens to Which We're Most Commonly Exposed

Some xenoestrogens are particularly known to promote cancer and sterilization. Researchers at Tufts Medical School in Boston found that a certain chemical detergent involved in plastic manufacturing stimulates breast cancer cell growth. This cancerous estrogenic compound (p-nonylphenol) belongs to a group of chemical compounds called phthalates, which are mainly used as plasticizers. These increase plastic flexibility—turning a hard plastic to a flexible plastic—and are often found in food containers, water bottles, children's toys, and commercial protein powder cans.

● ● ● **A correlation was found between heightened levels of estrogenic chemical residues in mothers and smaller penis size of their male children.**

Phthalates are also used in the manufacturing of foamed PVC, and they are commonly found in solvents, perfumes, pesticides, nail polish, adhesives, paint pigments, and lubricants. By 2004, manufacturers were producing about one billion pounds of phthalates each year. Phthalates were first produced in the 1920s and have been produced in large quantities since the 1950s, when PVC was introduced.

Studies on rodents involving large amounts of phthalates have shown damage to the liver, the kidneys, the lungs, and developing testes. A 2005 study reported that phthalates may mimic estrogen and cause feminization of baby boys (Barrett 2005).

Phthalates are some of the most dangerous chemicals in our world today. Researchers at the University of Missouri conducted studies in which urine samples from pregnant women in four states were collected. All the women were found to have substantial levels of phthalate residues in their urine.

● ● ● **Extra estrogen causes an increase in the size of estrogen-sensitive fatty tissues (such as belly fat); the enlarged fatty tissues produce more estrogen which induces even more fat gain.**

Another 2005 study revealed that upon birth of children from mothers with phthalate residues, there was a correlation between heightened levels of these estrogenic chemical residues and smaller penis size of their male children.

The evidence of the chemical-castrating effects of these xeno-estrogens is overwhelming, yet plastic remains one of the most common, cost-effective ingredients in many products that we routinely use. The manufacturers of plastics and pharmaceuticals do not favor changes in regulations. Not surprisingly, the studies have been criticized. They asserted that the media overstated the finding in the reports.

Xenoestrogens, Weight Gain, Obesity, and Syndrome X

Estrogen biosynthesis in humans occurs largely in the adipose tissues, which is where fat is stored. Adipose tissues produce the aromatase enzyme that synthesizes estrogen from the male androgen hormones. Estrogenic chemicals have shown the ability to bind to estrogen receptors and induce aromatase activity in fatty tissue, which increases estrogen levels and activity. This extra estrogen causes an increase in the size of estrogen-sensitive fatty tissues (such as belly fat). The enlarged fatty tissues produce more estrogen that induce even more fat gain, and so on and so forth.

● ● ● **There is a direct correlation between elevated estrogen and disorders involving obesity, blood sugar problems, elevated blood lipids, and high blood pressure.**

Obesity often involves disorders in blood sugar and hypertension, known as Syndrome X. For that matter, there is a direct correlation between elevated estrogen and disorders involving obesity, blood sugar problems, elevated blood lipids, and high blood pressure.

Researchers at the University of Texas-Galveston suggest that the current epidemic of obesity, diabetes, and hypertension may relate to chronic exposure to estrogenic chemicals. There are over a hundred thousand registered estrogenic chemicals which are currently used worldwide. Only a few of them are regulated in the United States. These substances promote benign and malignant tumors in men and women, and have shown the capacity to induce devastating sterilizing effects on various wildlife species and human reproductive functions. They are found in virtually every synthetic product that we use or consume.

Commonly Used Estrogenic Chemicals

- 4 MBC (sunscreen lotion)

- Hydroxy-anisole butyrate (food preservative)

- Atrazine (weed killer)

- Bisphenol-A (food preservative, plasticizer)

- Dieldrin (insecticide)

- DDT (insecticide, banned in the US but used in countries that export food to the US)

- Erythrosine (red dye 3)

- PCB (lubricants, adhesives, paints)

- P-nonylphenol (PVC, byproducts from detergents and spermicides)

- Parabens (lotions)

- Phthalates (plastic softeners)

Chapter 2

Phytoestrogens and Soy Isoflavones—Are They Part of the Problem or the Solution?

Phytoestrogens, also called plant estrogens, have been largely used to treat estrogen-related disorders and cancer. However, there is emerging evidence that some phytoestrogens may, in fact, do the opposite, and under certain conditions cause negative effects similar to estrogenic chemicals.

● ● ● **When there is an excess of estrogen in the body, any estrogen-promoting substance, whether chemical or natural, may be detrimental to one's health.**

Phytoestrogens occur naturally in many plants. They have structural and functional similarities to the human hormone estradiol. The most commonly known phytoestrogens are isoflavones, which are found in a variety of vegetables, grains, and legumes. By far, the highest amount of these isoflavones is found in soybeans. Other plant compounds with reported estrogenic properties include lignans, coumestans, and lactones. Isoflavones belong to a large group of polyphenolic compounds called flavonoids. Although many flavonoids are often called phytoestrogens, only a limited number have the potency to bind to estrogen receptors and promote estrogenic activity. Flavonoids often occur in mixtures of estrogen promoters and estrogen inhibitors. Some flavonoids such as chrysin (passion flower) and apigenine (chamomile) have shown the ability to inhibit estrogen activity, whereas others such as the soy isoflavone genistein were found to promote estrogen activity.

Flavonoids are known to have widely diverse beneficial biological effects, such as anti-inflammatory, antioxidant, antiviral, and anti-cancerous. Nonetheless, some flavonoids also modulate the functions and metabolism of sex hormones. It is this last property of flavonoids that can either improve or devastate the hormonal balance in the human body.

In times when overwhelming amounts of estrogenic chemicals are penetrating our environment in products, food, and water, it is critically important to know the difference between estrogen promoters and estrogen inhibitors. When there is an excess of estrogen in the body, any estrogen-promoting substance, whether chemical or natural, may be detrimental to one's health. There are currently large varieties of commercial products containing phytoestrogens that claim to help treat hormonal imbalance, estrogen disorders, menopausal symptoms, and cancer. The most popular of these are soy products and soy isoflavones supplements.

Most studies on soy are sponsored by grants from soy product manufacturers. Consequently, large parts of the current database that we find on soy are positive about the beneficial properties of soybeans. However, even though less advertised, there are also studies that provide substantial evidence about the harmful effects of soy and its related isoflavones. Soy is a cheap commodity that generates multibillion-dollar profits to soy product manufacturers worldwide. Facing the current popularity of soy as a source of protein and its wide application as a medicinal substance, it is very likely that the following information may appear as highly controversial. Nonetheless, the information is based on real studies that should not be overlooked.

How Soy Isoflavones Affect the Body

Soy isoflavones have been a dietary component for certain populations for many centuries. The consumption of soy has been generally considered to be beneficial. Epidemiological studies over the last decades have suggested that soy isoflavones may provide protective effects against breast, endometrial, and prostate cancer. Soy protein and soy isoflavones are major ingredients in a large variety of health and weight-loss products. However, recent studies raise serious concerns regarding soy. There is growing evidence that soy may not be as beneficial as it initially appeared to be. In fact, some studies suggest that soy isoflavones may harm the human body in the same manner as do xenoestrogens. There is also evidence that soy isoflavones may further accelerate the already existing harmful effects of xenoestrogens.

● ● ●   **Some studies suggest that soy isoflavones may harm the human body in the same manner as xenoestrogens.**

In one recent study, researchers concluded that soy isoflavones should not be used therapeutically to treat estrogen-related disorders and that more studies are needed to determine the real-life consequences of their estrogenic effects on the human body.

However, in spite of the conflicting evidence regarding soy, the same researchers still suggested that soy is safe. Not surprisingly, they also acknowledged that their review was sponsored by grants from the United Soybean Board, an association of soybean growers.

To understand how soy isoflavones affect the body, we first need to learn about their different forms and bioactivity. As you'll soon see, some soy isoflavones are highly bioactive, whereas others are not. Most important is the realization that the body recognizes the highly bioactive form of soy isoflavones as harmful toxins that need to be neutralized and eliminated.

Dietary sources of soybeans generally contain a mixture of three isoflavones: genistein, daidzein, and glycitein. These three isoflavones appear in two forms: free-aglycones isoflavones and conjugated (bound) isoflavones. Coumestrol also has been identified as a soy isoflavone, though in lower concentrations than the other isoflavones.

● ● ● **Soy isoflavones may accelerate the already existing harmful effects of estrogenic chemicals and, for that matter, may also contribute to estrogen-related disorders and increased risk for cancer.**

The biological activity of soy isoflavones depends on their chemical form. Free soy isoflavones (aglycones) are more readily absorbed than conjugated isoflavones. In order to be absorbed, isoflavones must be first digested and hydrolyzed into free aglycones. In their natural occurring state, isoflavones exist as glycosides, acetylglycosides, or malonyl glycosides. Following ingestion, the acetyl and malonyl chains are metabolized to genistein and daidzein, which are then hydrolyzed in the large intestines by gut bacteria, resulting in the production of their respective free-form aglucones, which, as noted, are highly absorbable.

Now here comes the interesting part: following absorption of the free isoflavones aglycones, the liver recognizes them as harmful substances that must be neutralized and eliminated, the same as chemical toxins. The isoflavones aglycones are then conjugated in the liver to glucuronic acid and sulfate. Once they're conjugated, they are treated as a waste product. Ninety percent of circulating isoflavones in the body are conjugated to glucuronic acid. Nonetheless, this natural process of neutralization in the liver may present additional problems. Glucuronic acid is a final product of a critically important metabolic pathway in the liver—the glucuronic acid pathway, which is responsible for the transport, metabolism, and neutralization of steroid hormones and their derivatives including estrogenic substances. Glucuronic acid is an expensive commodity in the body, with a limited supply that generally declines due to high metabolic stress, high levels of toxicity, and aging.

Apparently, a high intake of soy isoflavones may rob the liver from its pool of glucuronic acid, leaving it vulnerable to the ongoing assault of other environmental and endogenous estrogens. Thus, soy isoflavones may accelerate the already existing harmful effects of estrogenic chemicals and, for that matter, may also contribute to estrogen-related disorders and increased risk for cancer.

Furthermore, the liver, which has a limited capacity to neutralize toxins, can be overstressed by the overwhelming combination of xenoestrogens, phytoestrogens, and endogenous estrogens, and thus may fail to perform its normal duties. Under such conditions of excess estrogen and a stressed liver, one may be prone to suffer from estrogen-related disorders, fat gain, blood sugar disorders, hypertension, cardiovascular disease, and cancer.

Metabolic Profile and Safety of Soy

Due to the structural similarity to endogenous estrogen, there has been considerable research on the effects of soy isoflavones on endocrine functions in humans. A direct correlation was found between soy isoflavone intake and increased levels of circulating estradiol.

● ● ● **Progesterone is an "anti-estrogenic" hormone that helps balance estrogenic activity in the body.**

In a controlled diet study on women, Cassidy et al. reported a significant increase in plasma estradiol in women who consumed 60 g of soy protein (containing 45 mg isoflavones) per day. Subsequent studies found similar effects. Soy isoflavones were also found to delay peak progesterone concentrations in subjects consuming only 25–28 mg of soy isoflavones per day.

Progesterone is an "anti-estrogenic" hormone that helps balance estrogenic activity in the body. Any substance that suppresses progesterone would leave the body vulnerable to excess estrogen. Low progesterone levels are associated with estrogen disorders and aging in women.

Soy isoflavones have also shown disturbing effects on men's hormonal balance. Epidemiological evidence from the Takayama Study (Japan) suggested an inverse association between serum testosterone levels and soy consumption in Japanese men (Nagata 2000). Other studies showed no effect. However, all other studies were short-term and therefore inconclusive.

Soy and Infant Development

The adverse effects of soy isoflavones are even more pronounced in infants. There have been preliminary reports that isoflavones are excreted through breast milk. Irvine et al. hypothesized that infants may be more sensitive to the estrogenic effects of soy isoflavones due to low concentration of estrogen in their bodies.

In a controlled study at the University of Iowa, researchers found that women who had been exposed to soy-based formula during infancy would be more prone to suffer from a longer duration of menstrual bleeding and discomfort during menstruation, compared to women who were fed cow milk formula during infancy.

More disturbing is the effect of infant soy formula on the thyroid hormone. Deficiency of thyroid hormone is known to produce goiters in humans and has been reported in infants receiving exclusively soy-based diets. Low thyroid in infants is often associated with stunted growth. A study by Divi et al. (1997) indicated that the unconjugated form of genistein and daidzein isolated from soy protein was found to inhibit thyroid peroxidase, an enzyme involved in thyroid hormone synthesis. Another study featured a case report in which a male infant receiving a soy-based formula was diagnosed with congenital hypothyroidism. Even thyroxine (thyroide hormone drug) treatment failed to improve his condition—until the infant's diet was changed to cow's milk.

Soy isoflavones have also demonstrated adverse effects on reproductive function and development in animal studies. Estrogen-like effects have been observed in mice at high doses of soy isoflavones. In rats, male reproductive development and mating were reported to be adversely affected by exposure to dietary soy isoflavones.

Soy and Carcinogenicity

There is evidence that soy isoflavones may induce mutagenic and genetic toxicity. Anderson et al. reported that genistein and daidzein have the ability to increase the incidence of broken DNA strands in human sperm and peripheral lymphocytes. Even though common opinion considers the genotoxic potential of soy isoflavones as negligible, studies suggest the opposite.

Recognizing the mutagenic effects of soy isoflavones, Alfred et al. suggested, for the sake of safety, that there is a threshold level of dietary genistein, below which no increase in estrogen-dependent tumor is observed. Studies in animals showed that administration of genistein to mice produced significant increases in uterine weight and abnormal proliferation of the oviduct cells.

● ● ● **In one study, it was reported that prolonged consumption of soy-based diets had a stimulatory effect on proliferation of breast epithelium cells of premenopausal women.**

The cancer-promoting effects of isoflavones have been also observed in humans. McMichael-Philips et al. reported a significant increase in the proliferation rate of breast epithelium cells in premenopausal women with benign or malignant breast cancer who consumed 60 g of soy protein per day (45 mg of soy isoflavones per day). In another one-year study, Petrakis et al. reported that prolonged consumption of soy-based diets had a stimulatory effect on proliferation of breast epithelium cells of premenopausal women. Additionally, in vitro studies found stimulation of growth in human breast cancer cells in postmenopausal women.

These studies contradict other studies that found no correlation between soy consumption and breast cancer in postmenopausal women. Nonetheless, due to the conflicting evidence regarding soy isoflavones and how they affect cancer, it is important to present both sides and let individuals make their choices accordingly.

Soy and Hormonal Replacement Therapy

Soy isoflavones have been largely used as a natural alternative for hormone replacement therapy (HRT). However, there are contradictory reports in this category as well. Soy isoflavones have shown to help lower hot flash incidence by 40% (Albertazzi et al. 1998). Contrary to the above, Quella et al. reported that soy isoflavones were not effective in treating menopausal symptoms in a study of 177 breast cancer survivors. A conclusion to the effects of soy isoflavones as a replacement for HRT has not yet been reached.

Soy and Cardiovascular Functions

There are conflicting reports about the effect of soy isoflavones on the cardiovascular system. Recent studies reported a significant increase in blood urea nitrogen waste in women consuming soy protein, compared with a control diet. Nitrogen waste is known to adversely affect nitric oxide production and therefore impair vasodilation, while increasing levels of free radicals, which can damage blood vessels.

Soy isoflavones have also been regarded as a cholesterol-lowering agent. Nonetheless, studies state that based on the contradictory results of a limited number of studies, confirmation of the effects of soy isoflavones on serum cholesterol cannot yet be made.

Soy and Cognitive Functions

It is commonly believed that Japanese people are healthier, slower to age, and live longer than American people. The superior health state of Japanese people has been attributed to their high intake of dietary soy. However, recent studies revealed that the high consumption of soy may actually have adverse effects on them.

A cohort study of Seattle, Washington, Japanese-American men and women indicated that consumers of high amounts of tofu had lower cognitive function scores at baseline. Also, an association between tofu intake in midlife and reduced cognitive functions, as well as structural changes in the brain, was reported in Japanese-American males.

There are conflicting reports on the effects of soy intake on cognitive functions. Some reports support the notion that Japanese are less prone to suffer from age-related brain disease. White et al. (1996) found that the prevalence of Alzheimer's disease was lower in Japan that in Hawaii. Nonetheless, there isn't any conclusive correlation between these findings and soy intake, compared to previous findings that reported an inverse correlation between soy intake and cognitive function in Japanese people.

Summary

Studies investigating the metabolic effects of soy isoflavones indicate that they're readily absorbed and exert estrogenic activity similar to the human hormone estradiol. Due to conflicting reports on the effects of soy isoflavones on humans, more studies are needed to reach conclusive evidence as to the estrogenic mechanisms of soy isoflavones. Until then, soy and soy isoflavones should not be used therapeutically to treat menopausal symptoms and estrogen-related disorders. Furthermore, due to the current ongoing assault of xenoestrogens in the environment, food, and water, any estrogen-promoting substance, including soy, may contribute to the problem instead of the solution.

Phytoestrogens in Food, Spices, and Herbs— Harmful vs. Beneficial

● ◗ ● **Any substance that promotes estrogen and suppresses progesterone may contribute to the problem of excess estrogen in the body.**

A large variety of phytoestrogens besides soy isoflavones are found in food, spices, and herbs. Some of them are common ingredients in traditional herbal remedies, and are also used today as alternatives for treating estrogen disorders, menopausal symptoms, and cancer. Studies, however, show that not all phytoestrogens are the same. Recent findings reveal that the different phytoestrogens have different effects on estrogen receptors (ER). Some show estrogen-promoting effects, whereas others have been found to work as estrogen inhibitors. Virtually all phytoestrogens were found to be either neutral or antagonistic to progesterone. Overall, certain phytoestrogens may be harmful, whereas others may be beneficial.

Estrogen-Promoting Herbs

Recent studies at the Cancer Research Division of the California Public Health Foundation in Berkeley found that the most potent and estrogen receptors-binding products were soy milk, licorice, and red clover. Licorice and red clover (both in the leguminosae family) also showed potent progesterone-inhibiting properties. The estrogen-promoting and progesterone-suppressing effects of these herbs should raise serious concerns. As noted, any substance that promotes estrogen and suppresses progesterone may contribute to the problem of excess estrogen in the body.

In 1940, there was an incidence where red clover was found to cause some devastating effects on the reproductive functions of herds of merino sheep in Australia. Studies described this phenomenon as "clover disease." The phytoestrogen formononetin in red clover was determined to be the main cause for the reproductive impairments and near-extinction of this clover-fed herd of Australian sheep.

Other herbs that were found to activate estrogen receptors are dong gui, damiana, black cohosh, verbena, and motherwort. Their active extracts have shown the capacity to bind to estrogen receptors and stimulate cell proliferation.

Commercial black cohosh extract has an extensive clinical history in Western Europe for relief of menopausal symptoms, which are commonly associated with estrogen deficiency. The notable estrogenic effect of black cohosh may help treat menopausal symptoms; however, there are also disturbing reports on the cancer-promoting effects of this herb in women who already suffer from breast cancer. Other reports indicate liver-damaging effects of black cohosh after long-term use.

Anti-estrogenic Herbs

Certain herbs have shown the capacity to antagonize estrogen receptors or inhibit estrogen. Researchers have found that certain flavonoids such as green tea polyphenols and quercetin (found in onion and garlic) have shown anti-estrogenic, anti-proliferative activity when in high concentrations.

Studies also have found that combinations of resveratrol (found in red wine and grapes), apigenine (found in chamomile), and quercetin demonstrated substantial anti-cancerous effects on tumor growth, but only apigenine and quercetin showed anti-metastatic effects.

Other herbs that have shown anti-proliferative properties are mandrake, juniper, and mistletoe, all of which were found to inhibit cell proliferation in both ER+ and ER– breast cancer cell lines. Since those contain phytoestrogens, researchers implied that their growth inhibitory mechanism of action is not likely to be estrogen regulated. Some of these herbs have an extensive history of use as herbal therapies for treatment of cancer.

Anti-estrogenic Spices

Phytoestrogens are found in spices including thyme, oregano, and turmeric. However, there is substantial evidence that some of these herbs may actually antagonize estrogen receptors, and therefore, could be highly beneficial as estrogen inhibitors and anti-cancerous nutrients.

Thyme and oregano have been used since biblical times as spices and remedies. They're highly notable for their antiviral, antibacterial, and detoxifying properties. For that matter, they are highly beneficial in supporting liver detoxification, and thereby help promote neutralization of estrogenic substances. There is no evidence that thyme and oregano induce any estrogenic effect on the body.

Turmeric is a spice commonly used in Middle Eastern, Mediterranean, and Indian foods. Curcumin, the active ingredient in turmeric (and curry) exhibited multiple suppressive effects on breast carcinoma cells. Studies in India and China revealed that curcumin's anti-cancerous effects are induced by antagonizing both ER+ and ER– cells. Researchers concluded that curcumin isoflavones could also be used to inhibit the estrogenic effects of pesticides and environmental xenoestrogens.

Estrogen-Promoting Spices

Contrary to oregano, thyme, and turmeric, there are spices that actually promote estrogen, the most notable of which are licorice and hops. Studies revealed that all kinds of licorice are estrogenic. Hops is an ingredient in beer that gives the drink its unique bitter taste. Anecdotal reports claim that women harvesting hops often begin menstruation within two days of the beginning of the harvest. Studies have identified phytoestrogens in hops extracts. It is very likely that the typical "beer belly" may be related to excess estrogenic activity in the body due to binge drinking.

 **It is very likely that the typical beer belly may be related to excess estrogenic activity in the body due to binge drinking.**

Summary

It becomes evidently clear that when the right choices of food, spices, and herbs are made, applications of natural anti-estrogenic compounds may have preventive and therapeutic effects against tumors induced by estrogenic chemicals.

Researchers at Tufts University, School of Medicine, Boston, Massachusetts, reported that many estrogenic chemicals have been found to stimulate the growth of estrogen receptors positive (ER+) breast cancer cells. The therapeutic use of natural compounds that inhibit ER+ breast cancer cells could be highly effective.

Nonetheless, more studies are needed to elucidate the beneficial or harmful effects of phytoestrogens, in particular those that are commonly found in our food, spices, and herbs. Due to the conflicting evidence regarding the estrogenic effects of phytoestrogens, there is much confusion today as to what is beneficial and what is harmful. It is therefore important to establish a conclusive database of what are estrogen-promoting substances and what are estrogen-inhibiting substances.

Conclusion

As a final note, let's briefly summarize the correlation between xeno-estrogens and phytoestrogens and how their combination affects our health

Today we face an ever-growing ecological problem due to the ongoing invasion of estrogenic chemicals to our environment, soil, products, food, and water. There is growing evidence that estrogen-promoting phytoestrogens may accelerate the problem, whereas estrogen-inhibiting phytoestrogens may actually be part of the solution. Just to put things in perspective: in general, phytoestrogens are thought to wash out of the body within several days, in contrast to the months or years that xenoestrogens take to be excreted.

For that matter, any viable solution for xenoestrogens must incorporate a daily nutritional regiment based on anti-estrogenic foods, spices, herbs, and extracts—all in sufficient amounts. Estrogenic chemicals invade our bodies like heavy war machines. We require plenty of anti-estrogenic nutrients—soldiers if you will—to effectively combat, neutralize, and render them inactive within the body.

Chapter 3

Redefining the Term "Diet"

Why Most Current Diets Are Doomed to Fail

Most diets used today fail because they violate one basic survival principle—the survival of every species depends on its ability to live and eat in accordance with its primal genetic makeup. This is the law of nature.

● ◐ ● **We cannot survive well on foods that don't fit our genes.**

Each species has its own specific biological needs. You never see a cat eating cucumbers, nor a rabbit eating meat—but what about humans?

Unfortunately, we're the only species on this planet that has chosen to eat fake food, food that doesn't fit our genes. People today habitually use artificial sweeteners instead of natural fruits or grain sweeteners; eat imitation cheese made from processed soy instead of fresh organic dairy; use synthetic flavoring instead of natural plant extracts; and add chemical preservatives instead of natural antioxidants.

The human body has never adapted to such a chemical insult. Quite simply, we cannot survive well on food that doesn't fit our genes.

Food and Survival

Scientists believe that our survival on this planet depended on the capacity to adapt to environmental factors and foods that existed over 10,000 years ago. This adaptation process is still deeply carved in our genes.

According to the thrifty genes theory, we carry today the same genes as our ancestors, the late Paleolithic cavemen, but the world that we live in today is very different from theirs. The food that we eat now is not the same as the food that humans adapted to millenniums ago. Many popular food items, including so-called "healthy" foods, virtually don't fit our genes.

In a recent review in the *Journal of Applied Physiology,* researchers suggested that the main cause for the current epidemic of obesity, diabetes, cardiovascular disease, and cancer may relate to the failure of current diet to adequately fit our primal genetic makeup.

● ◍ ● **Our bodies must be nourished with food that actually fits our genes.**

Even though food is more accessible than ever, much of it does not fully satisfy the body's real biological needs. Besides being chemically loaded or fake, today's foods are often highly processed and therefore nutritionally deficient. Men and women alike are being chronically deprived of certain critical nutrients that would have otherwise provided them with the means to better survive, while sustaining a lean, healthy, and functional body.

Along with this view, scientists believe that due to the disappearance of these critical nutrients from our diet, certain positive phenotypes (properties) of genes—responsible for keeping us alive—are constantly inhibited. This then causes the over-expression of negative phenotypes, which are responsible for obesity, metabolic disorders, and chronic diseases. If we don't take action to change our diets, we will continue to become fatter and unhealthier. Apparently, if we are not actively surviving, we are passively dying.

This all leads to one conclusion: to maintain primal health, our bodies require more than just any vitamins, minerals, antioxidants, protein, fat, and carbs. Our bodies must be nourished with food that actually fits our genes. For that matter, our bodies must be provided with additional nutrients that help support and modulate the hormonal system, thereby protecting us against metabolic decline and aging. Our bodies have been genetically pre-programmed to be nourished and protected in this way.

Redefining the Term "Diet"

The solution to this nutritional problem requires the means to bring back the missing nutrients and provide the body with food that fits our genes, food to which we have primarily adapted.

Most Estrogenic Diets Today

Many of us aren't aware of the fact that a large part of the food that we eat is highly estrogenic. Many people also consume a lot of alcohol, which is known for its estrogen-promoting effect. This ever-growing problem is further accelerated by many of today's popular diets.

Most notable are the so-called "high-protein–low-carb" diets. Diets in this category promote a high consumption of commercial meats and dairy, which are often loaded with hormones and chemical preservatives. To make matters worse, low-carb products are often made with soy protein, petroleum-based sweeteners, and sugar alcohol, all of which contribute to excess estrogen in the body.

Statistically, those on a low-carb diet are prone to suffer from a fat-gain rebound, often regaining more weight than they initially lost. This weight fluctuation may relate to the high prevalence of excess estrogenic substances in low-carb diets.

Other current popular diets, whether the Zone, South Beach, Atkins, or the Blood Type diet, all fail to fully address the problem of excess estrogen, and don't offer any solutions. Consequently, people today have no idea what to do. In spite of being on more diets than ever, people in this country are becoming even fatter and less healthy.

The Anti-Estrogenic Approach

The solution for excess estrogen, and the weight gain and disorders it can cause, requires the incorporation of anti-estrogenic foods and supplements. (This also requires taking proactive measures such as

The principles of human nutrition should be redefined as follows:

1. **Go down on the food chain.**

   Early foods such as fruits, vegetables, legumes, roots, nuts, seeds, fertile eggs, wild-catch marine food, and raw, fresh dairy would most likely fit our genetic makeup better than the later post-agricultural foods such as grains, sugar, overfed farm animals, and refined, processed, or chemically loaded food.

2. **Minimize the intake of chemically loaded conventional food.**

   Eat organic food if possible. Minimize intake of synthetic vitamins.

3. **Supplement your body with hormonal-supportive nutrients.**

   Due to soil depletion, industrial harvesting, and food processing methods, there are substantial deficiencies of critically important hormonal-supportive nutrients in our diets. Our actual survival may depend on these missing nutrients. One cannot overlook these facts today when hormonal imbalance, and in particular, excess estrogen-related disorders, are at an all-time high.

liver detoxification and exercise.) The following is a brief description of anti-estrogenic elements.

Anti-estrogenic Food

Anti-estrogenic food is any food that helps inhibit or counteract excess estrogen and its adverse effects. For that matter, the term "anti-estrogenic" describes food that either helps inhibit estrogen or beneficially modulates its metabolism, promoting anti-estrogenic hormones such as progesterone in women and testosterone in men.

Liver Detoxification

The benefits of the anti-estrogenic dietary approach can be substantially enhanced by proactive measures such as liver detox. The liver is the site for estrogen metabolism. When it is strained or overwhelmed by chemical toxins or by estrogenic substances in food, it may fail to properly metabolize and neutralize estrogen. That can lead to an excess of harmful circulating estrogens such as the alpha 16-hydroxy estrogens associated with weight gain, bloating, metabolic disorders, and cancer.

Liver detox via special foods, spices, and herbal applications can help provide the body with the power and means to metabolize estrogen and sustain a healthy hormonal balance.

Exercise

A critical part of being proactive in the war against excess estrogen is exercise. It is now known that exercise lowers estrogen levels in men and women. Researchers have found that exercise and fat loss are in fact anti-estrogenic. According to Dr. Mark Mattson (2005), professor of neuroscience at Johns Hopkins University, women who lose fat tend to be consequently more physically active in a particular manner. While getting leaner and stronger, due to increased physical activity, they also show a dramatic decrease in estrogen levels.

● ● ● **A critical part of being proactive in the war against excess estrogen is getting exercise.**

It is very likely that fat loss and physical exercise trigger survival mechanisms that promote energy expenditure and improved fuel utilization during extreme conditions that require fight-or-flight activities. Nature may protect women from the extra responsibility of having babies during hard times that involve danger and physical or mental stress. And it does so by lowering estrogen levels, making women leaner, stronger, and virtually addicted to physical exercise and ready to fight or flee to better survive. Lower estrogen levels are also associated with a lower risk for cancer.

Fat loss and exercise affect men in a similar manner. Physically active, lean men were found to have higher ratios of testosterone to estrogen than overweight sedentary men. Obese men were found to suffer from the highest levels of circulating estrogen, also associated with a lower capacity to resist fatigue, stress, and disease.

Apparently, nutrition and exercise that lower estrogen and burn body fat are also associated with higher survival capabilities.

Elimination of Estrogenic Food and Chemicals

The solution for excess estrogen requires the virtual elimination of estrogen-promoting foods and chemicals from the diet.

Eating organic is a major step ahead. Nonetheless, some conventional foods are safer than others. For example, fruits and vegetables that are peeled for consumption, such as avocado and bananas, are safer than those with an edible peel, such as berries and apples. Also, dairy products, including protein shakes, should be manufactured without chemicals and hormones and be pesticide-free. Note that wild-catch fish and dairy from grass-fed cows are superior to their conventional equivalents.

Chapter 4

The Program

The most effective way to fight excess estrogen is to combine anti-estrogenic food with estrogen-inhibiting herbs. Plant estrogen inhibitors should be added to the diet in a pure, isolated, or highly standardized form to maximize their inhibitory potency, and to prevent potential counter-effects of naturally occurring estrogen-promoting compounds. Adding these estrogen inhibitors to the diet is the only viable way to grant optimum assimilation. It is practically impossible to consume the essential raw herbs in the large amounts that are often required for effective estrogenic inhibition. Passionflower, for instance, is very bitter, hard to digest, and almost nauseating in its raw form. The isolation of the active inhibiting compound makes it more edible and easily assimilated.

● ● ● **The diet offers clear priorities as to what comes first and what comes second—what foods work and what do not.**

● ● ● **The most effective way to fight excess estrogen is to combine anti-estrogenic foods with plant-estrogen inhibitors.**

Making the Program Simple

One of the main reasons for failure to stick with a diet is over-complexity. There are too many restrictions and impracticalities including calorie counting, restriction of carbs or fat, measuring the ratio between protein, carbs, and fat, and carrying around obscure food charts. The human diet should not be that complicated.

The Anti-Estrogenic Diet is based on a solid principle and a simple solution. The program reintroduces anti-estrogenic foods together with plant estrogen inhibitors, while eliminating estrogen-promoting foods and chemicals.

Overall, the Anti-Estrogenic Diet offers clear priorities as to what foods work and what foods do not. The program consists of three lines of nutritional defense against excess estrogen. These lines of nutritional defense are literally the most critical elements of the diet. Any other elements, such as eating low fat or low carb, may be important at times, but nevertheless they are secondary to the real issue. Without these critical lines of defense, the body may not be able to resist the ever-growing onslaught of excess estrogen due to chemicals, drugs, and aging.

The First Line of Nutritional Defense Against Excess Estrogen

Cruciferous Vegetables, Citrus Fruits, Omega-3 Oil, Organic Dairy, and Estrogen Inhibitors

The first line of nutritional defense against excess estrogen consists of the most important anti-estrogenic foods and the most potent plant estrogen inhibitors. It incorporates cruciferous vegetables, citrus fruits, omega-3 oil-rich foods (flaxseed, hempseed, and their derived oils), as well as wild-catch fatty fish. Also included are organic dairy products, in particular, those derived from whole milk (such as butter and aged cheese). Note that dairy may be problematic for some people and, therefore, should be treated cautiously (see Chapter 5). For best results, the foods from this list should be combined with highly standardized or isolated plant estrogen inhibitors in a supplemental form derived from passionflower, chamomile flower, and cruciferous vegetables.

This first line of nutritional defense incorporates foods that have a proven capacity to directly interfere with estrogen metabolism, helping induce an anti-estrogenic effect on the body. Nonetheless, the foods listed below in the Second and Third Lines of Nutritional Defense are as important, and can further contribute to the reversal of related metabolic disorders, fat loss, and lowering of the risk of cancer in both women and men. In summary, all three lines of defense are critically important for the overall success of the Anti-Estrogenic Diet.

The Second Line of Nutritional Defense Against Excess Estrogen
Plant Sterol-Rich Foods—Nuts, Seeds, Avocado, Olives, Stabilized Rice Germ Oil, and Stabilized Wheat Germ Oils

The second line of nutritional defense against excess estrogen consists of foods that promote the anti-estrogenic hormones—progesterone in women and testosterone in men. The most important foods in this category are raw nuts and seeds. In addition there are also other viable plant-derived sterol-rich foods, such as avocado and olives, stabilized rice germ, stabilized wheat germ, as well as their cold-press oils. All of these foods are rich in plant sterols. Nuts, seeds, avocados, and olives are rich in omega-9 mono-unsaturated oil, which is relatively stable, safe, and non-estrogenic.

● ● ● *Note that nuts and seeds should not be combined with any grains or sugar. These naturally high-fat foods work better in a low glycemic environment. They combine well with vegetables and protein foods.*

Nuts and seeds were introduced to the human body long before grains. It is very likely that our bodies have better adapted primarily to the low-glycemic fat fuel coming from nuts and seeds, than to our modern higher-glycemic carb fuel that comes from grains or processed sugars.

The Third Line of Defense Against Excess Estrogen

Liver Detoxifiers—Green Vegetables, Fruits, Spices, and Herbs

The third line of defense against excess estrogen consists of food items that work as co-factors—enhancing the anti-estrogenic effect of the foods and herbs previously listed above in the First and Second Lines of Defense). Furthermore, this list is comprised of foods, spices, and herbs that provide all essential nutrients and also promote liver detoxification. This includes all green vegetables, fruits (such as citrus, all kinds of berries, apple, papaya, and pineapple), legumes (excluding soy), whole oats, and barley that provide the body with critical compounds called proteoglucans (known for lowering cholesterol and stabilizing blood sugar). Other important contributors for liver detox and the overall defense against excess estrogen are the spices turmeric, oregano, thyme, rosemary, and sage, as well as herbs such as milk thistle, dandelion root, shilijit, amla berries, ginger, and gotukola.

Liver detox is critically important to the neutralization of estrogenic chemicals and metabolites. It also helps facilitate a metabolic environment that favors fat burning and energy production. Fat burning is an anti-estrogenic activity. The reduction in the size of fatty tissues is associated with the lowering of estrogen levels.

● ● ● **It is important to note that the most important of the aforementioned foods are *green vegetables,* which are ubiquitous in the Anti-Estrogenic Diet. They should be incorporated *every day* to enhance the overall nourishing and anti-estrogenic effect of the diet.**

Liver detox and its related fat breakdown can be dramatically enhanced by periodic fasting or under-eating, in particular during the stressful active hours of the day. Undereating, when based on liver detoxifying foods alone, can help lower the metabolic stress on the liver, accelerate the removal of toxins, and enhance the liver's capacity to neutralize excess estrogen.

Exercise

Scientists believe that Homo sapiens are programmed to be physically active. There is a growing amount of evidence to the fact that exercise is programmed in our genes. The question is not how beneficial exercise is, but rather how much damage will the body incur without it?

There is indeed a direct correlation between an inactive lifestyle and many modern diseases. Studies have found that a lack of physical activity can adversely trigger negative phenotypes of genes, responsible for severe metabolic disorders including insulin resistance, hypertension, and obesity. Exercise can help reverse this problem by triggering positive phenotypes of genes, responsible for stabilizing blood sugar, lowering blood pressure, and burning fat.

When incorporated with anti-estrogenic foods and supplements, exercise can effectively facilitate fat loss, lower estrogen levels, and counteract its adverse effects.

First Line of Nutritional Defense

ANTI-ESTROGENIC FOODS:

- Cruciferous vegetables

- Citrus fruits

- Omega-3 oils (flaxseeds, hempseeds)

- Wild-catch fatty fish

- Organic dairy (moderate servings)

ESTROGEN INHIBITORS—HERBS (IN EXTRACT):

- Passionflower

- Chamomile flower

- Cruciferous indoles

Second Line of Nutritional Defense

FOODS THAT PROMOTE ANTI-ESTROGENIC HORMONES
PROGESTERONE (WOMEN) AND TESTOSTERONE (MEN):

- Raw nuts and seeds

- Avocado

- Olives and their cold-pressed oil

- Stabilized rice germ oil

- Stabilized wheat germ oil

Third Line of Nutritional Defense

FOODS THAT WORK AS CO-FACTORS AND PROMOTE LIVER
DETOXIFICATION:

- Green vegetables

- Fruits (citrus, berries, apples, papaya, pineapple)

- Whole oats and barley

- Legumes (other than soy)

- Spices (turmeric, oregano, thyme, rosemary, and sage)

- Herbs (i.e., milk thistle, dandelion root, shilijit, amla berries, ginger, and gotukola)

Chapter 5

Anti-Estrogenic Foods and Estrogen Inhibitors

Anti-estrogenic foods are easily accessible and can be found in groceries, supermarkets, and health-food stores. However, plant-derived estrogen inhibitors aren't so easily accessible and require special attention to their sourcing, quality, standardization, and potency. Nonetheless, the combination of anti-estrogenic food with estrogen inhibitors is the best way to counteract excess estrogen.

Anti-Estrogenic Foods
Cruciferous Vegetables

Most important anti-estrogenic foods are the cruciferous vegetables such as broccoli, cauliflower, brussels sprouts, and cabbage. The estrogen-inhibiting and modulating effects of cruciferous indoles may explain why crucifers have been widely regarded as a cancer-preventing food.

The active ingredients in crucifers—indole 3 carbinol, DIM, and indole 3 acetate—have shown substantial capacity to shift estrogen metabolism to produce beneficial antioxidant and anti-cancerous metabolites. Cruciferous indoles work as a first defense against excess estrogen. Studies reveal that cruciferous indoles can increase the ratio of beneficial estrogen metabolites (2-hydroxy estrogens) over harmful estrogen metabolites (16-hydroxy estrogens). It has been established that a high ratio of the chemicals 2-hydroxy to 16-hydroxy estrogens is associated with a low risk for estrogen-related cancer.

Onion and Garlic

Two other important anti-estrogenic foods are onion and garlic. In both, the active ingredient is the antioxidant flavonoid quercetin. Known for its immuno-supporting and liver-detoxifying properties, quercetin has also shown the capacity to inhibit the enzymes that synthesize estrogen when applied in high concentrations. Furthermore, quercetin works in synergy with other estrogen-inhibiting flavonoids to accelerate their overall anti-estrogenic effect in the body.

Omega-3 Oils

● ● ● **Plant sterols, found in raw nuts and seeds promote the anti-estrogenic hormones: progesterone in women and testosterone in men.**

Omega-3 oils, also known as N-3 oils, are essential to the body. They consist of long-chain polyunsaturated fatty acids and are derived from flaxseed, hempseed, or fatty fish such as salmon, tuna, mackerel, or sardines. Omega-3 oil has been found to be highly beneficial in modulating estrogen metabolism, with a critical balancing effect on excess estrogen. Omega-3 oils protect the body against the estrogen-promoting effects of omega-6 (N-6) vegetable oils, which when in excess, could increase the risk for estrogen dominance and estrogen-related cancer.

Nuts and Seeds

Nuts and seeds help fight excess estrogen by promoting anti-estrogenic hormones. Raw nuts and seeds are rich in certain fatty compounds called plant sterols, which help promote progesterone production in women and testosterone production in men. Both progesterone and testosterone work as anti-estrogenic hormones by counteracting estrogen and balancing its excess.

● ● ● **Estrogen dominance is believed to be responsible for age-related weight gain and metabolic disorders in both men and women.**

Aging and stress are associated with a substantial loss of progesterone in women and testosterone in men. The loss of these anti-estrogenic hormones causes estrogen dominance in both sexes. Estrogen dominance, with an excess of circulating estrogen, is believed to be responsible for the typical age-related weight gain and metabolic disorders in men and women. By virtue of their hormone-balancing properties, nuts and seeds help induce both anti-estrogenic and anti-aging effects. Researchers believe that nuts and seeds were a primal component of the human diet long before grains. Because of that, humans had a longer time to adapt and benefit from nuts and seeds as a source of nutrients and fuel.

Avocado, Olives, Oils, and Germs

Nuts and seeds aren't the only sterol-containing foods. There are hundreds of known plant sterols and most likely there are many more yet to be discovered. Besides supporting sex hormones, plant sterols have been found to have cholesterol-lowering properties. Scientists speculate that these cholesterol-like plant compounds may be one of the secret weapons to fight aging. Note that plant sterols can become rapidly rancid when reacting with oxygen, light, and heat. Therefore, it is highly recommended to incorporate a variety of fresh, plant-sterol-containing foods in their raw state. Samples of sterol-rich foods are avocados, olives, rice germ, wheat germ, whole oats, and their cold pressed oils.

Greens, Fruits, Spices, and Herbs

Fruits, greens, spices, and herbs provide nutrients that help detoxify the liver and thereby counteract estrogen.

Fruits such as oranges, grapefruit, berries, papaya, pineapple, kiwis, and apples provide the body with antioxidants, vitamins, enzymes, and co-factors that help protect the body from oxygen free radicals, while lowering the overall metabolic stress on the liver. Note that citrus fruits contain anti-estrogenic flavonones that have a mild anti-estrogenic effect, but nevertheless may be effective, if applied in large amounts.

Green leafy vegetables provide a large variety of phytonutrients that support the body's hormonal system, enzyme pool, and detoxifying power. Greens are a viable source for bioactive minerals, B vitamins, methyl groups, and phosphates, all of which enhance the liver's capacity to produce energy, remove toxins, and metabolize hormones—including estrogen.

Spices such as oregano, thyme, rosemary, sage, and turmeric are known for their antibacterial and antiviral properties. They also contain volatile oils that promote liver detox. Recent studies found that turmeric has anti-estrogenic and anti-cancerous properties. Turmeric has shown the capacity to antagonize and destroy estrogen receptor-positive (ER+) cancer cells, and thereby inhibit tumor growth. The anti-estrogenic effect of spices may relate to their capacity to work as potent co-factors with other compounds in protecting the body against excess estrogen.

Herbs such as milk thistle and dandelion root are known to be potent liver detoxifiers. Other beneficial herbs are shilajit, amla berries, ginger, and gotukola. These provide essential acids, trace minerals, and anti-oxidants as well as other nutritionally supportive compounds, all of which are anti-inflammatory, immuno-supportive, and liver-enhancing nutrients. As noted, the liver is the organ that metabolizes and neutralizes estrogen. For that matter, any liver detoxifier helps defend the body against excess estrogen.

Organic Dairy

Dairy has been a major component of human diets for thousands of years. There is emerging evidence that it is highly beneficial in more ways than one. Besides its superior nutritional composition of amino acids, minerals, and vitamins, dairy is also a viable source of anti-estrogenic nutrients.

Recent findings reveal that a certain fatty compound in dairy called conjugated linoleic acid (CLA) is both anti-estrogenic and anti-cancerous. CLA is found in milk fat, with the highest concentration in whole-milk products (such as aged cheese and butter) derived from grass-fed cows. CLA is also found in human mothers' milk. Statistically, high levels of CLA in breast milk are correlated with decreased incidence of cancer in both mothers and their children. Besides dairy, CLA occurs naturally (in smaller amounts) in grass-fed animals' fat.

● ● ● **Organic dairy products, particularly those made from grass-fed cows, provide the body with nutrients that have shown profound anti-estrogenic and anti-cancerous properties.**

A certain isomer in CLA (cis 9, trans 11) called rumenic acid, has shown a long-lasting impact on lowering the risk of mammary cancer in animals. Some scientists speculate that breast cancer may already be prevented in early life with a high intake of CLA.

Lab studies indicated that CLA has a profound fat-loss effect in animals. More studies are needed to elucidate whether CLA can induce similar effects in humans. Nonetheless, there is evidence that CLA may help prevent fat gain.

There are also some reports that indicated adverse effects of CLA on insulin sensitivity. However, these reports are based on isolated isomers of CLA. More studies are needed to investigate how CLA affects weight loss and insulin sensitivity. Nonetheless, as noted, there is profound evidence to CLA's anti-estrogenic and tumor suppressing effects.

Researchers also believe that the complex of CLA isomers, as it naturally occurs in dairy, may be superior to isolated isomers such as in commercial supplements. The researchers indicated that CLA isomers work similar to omega-3 oils, suppressing N-6 metabolism and their related estrogenic and growth-promoting effect on breast cancer cells.

● ● ●   **Estrogen inhibitors can help fight excess estrogen by interfering with its metabolism and virtually blocking its harmful effects.**

In conclusion, organic dairy products, particularly those made from grass-fed cows, provide the body with nutrients that have shown profound anti-estrogenic and anti-cancerous properties. Dairy is one of the most restricted foods among dieters, partly because of the common belief that dairy products are fattening, and partly because many people have sensitivities to dairy. Regardless, the anti-estrogenic and anti-cancerous properties of dairy are outstandingly beneficial, in particular today when the ever-growing assault of estrogenic chemicals is causing an epidemic of estrogen-related disorders and cancer in men, women, and children.

Notes

- In cases of insulin resistance or diabetes, it is highly advisable to cautiously regulate the serving size of dairy per meal and thereby avoid undesirable side effects.

- Not all dairy products are the same. While organic dairy has shown anti-estrogenic and anti-cancerous properties, conventional dairy, which often is loaded with estrogenic chemicals and hormones, may affect the body in the opposite way.

Estrogen Inhibitors

There is growing evidence that certain compounds in plants have a unique capacity to inhibit estrogen and—surprisingly—shift its metabolism to favor the production of antioxidant/anti-cancerous metabolites instead of harmful metabolites.

Summary

Crucifers, omega-3 oils, nuts, seeds, avocados, olives, stabilized rice germ oil, stabilized wheat germ oil, whole oats, and barley, greens, citrus fruits, berries, spices, herbs, and organic dairy provide the anti-estrogenic nutrients the body needs to win the battle against excess estrogen and its related weight gain and disorders.

When in excess, estrogen and its harmful metabolites (16-hydroxy estrogens) promote fat gain, disorders, and cancer. Estrogen inhibitors can help fight excess estrogen by interfering with its metabolism and virtually blocking its harmful effects. Their supporting effects go far beyond those that we get from vitamins, minerals, and anti-oxidants.

Unfortunately, plant-derived estrogen inhibitors are often missing in our diets. While some of them actually appear in small amounts in our food, others are totally absent. Estrogen inhibitors are currently a topic of great interest by virtue of their potential benefits in fighting cancer.

In their natural state, estrogen inhibitors are generally countered by other compounds that actually promote estrogen. This leads researchers to believe that estrogen inhibitors must be isolated from the plant into a highly standardized form in order to reach maximum inhibition potency. Furthermore, Dutch researchers have recently found that estrogen inhibitors possess a superior inhibition power when combined together.

Estrogen Inhibitors—where they're derived from

The estrogen inhibitors most deficient in our diets are the kinds of plant flavones that can be derived from the herbs passionflower and chamomile flower. Ironically, these missing inhibitors have also demonstrated the highest inhibition potency. More accessible are estrogen inhibiting flavones and flavonones found in garlic, onion, citrus fruits, raw honey, and bee products. Other accessible estrogen inhibiting compounds are indoles found in the cruciferous vegetables broccoli, cauliflower, brussels sprouts, and cabbage.

The following is a list of estrogen inhibitors—flavones, flavonones, and indoles:

List of Estrogen Inhibitors and Their Sources

ESTROGEN-INHIBITING FLAVONES AND FLAVONONES:

- Chrysin—passion flower—flavone
- Apigenine—chamomile—flavone
- Quercetin—onion, garlic, red apples, and grapes—flavone
- Naringenin—citrus—flavonone

ESTROGEN-INHIBITING INDOLES (ALL DERIVED FROM CRUCIFEROUS VEGETABLES):

- Indole 3 carbinol

- Diindolymethane (DIM)

- Indole 3 acetate

Estrogen Inhibitors—Co-factors

Certain nutrients can help support the actions of estrogen inhibitors by enhancing their inhibition potencies. These help detoxify the liver and stabilize blood sugar, thereby preventing undesirable insulin resistance-related fat gain, which is also associated with increased estrogen activity in the body.

Estrogen inhibitor co-factors include: nutrients in green vegetables; bioflavonoids which support estrogen-inhibiting flavones; antioxidants such as natural vitamin C (in amla berries); resveratrol (in red wine and grapes); green tea polyphenols; liver detoxifiers such as the amino acids methoine, cysteine, and taurine; ergogenics such as the amino acids lysine and carnitine; and blood sugar stabilizers such as turmeric, fenugreek, and shilijit.

Notes:

- Plant-derived estrogen inhibitors are not estrogen mimickers. Unlike soy isoflavones, they do not have any inherent estrogen activity.

- Plant estrogen inhibitors are not steroids. Their inhibition mechanisms are different than steroids. Unlike steroids, plant estrogen inhibitors are botanical extracts derived from plants that have traditionally been used to treat ailments and support the body's metabolism.

Chapter 6

The Program's Three-Week Jump-Start

The program's jump-start is based on three phases. Each phase lasts one week:

Phase I	**Liver Detox**	Week 1
Phase II	**High Fat**	Week 2
Phase III	**Reintroduction of Foods**	Week 3

The first two phases are the most restrictive; nevertheless, they're also the most anti-estrogenic and beneficial. The third phase gradually brings back restricted foods such as pasta, bread, and meat into the diet. However, this phase must be followed gradually and properly to avoid undesirable setbacks.

Even though the third phase may be seen as somewhat compromised in comparison to the first two phases, it is still critically important for the success of the diet in the long run. Once tried out, the third phase can be converted to a follow-up phase that can be modified to accommodate individual needs such as personal lifestyle, schedule, and food availability.

Chapter 7

Phase I:
Liver Detoxification

The goal of the first week is to maximize the removal of toxins from the liver. The liver is the site for estrogen metabolism as well as other critical functions including the regulation of lipids and glucose metabolism. Liver detox can help enhance liver functioning and create a metabolic environment that favors the utilization of fats and carbohydrates for energy. A healthy liver can grant a superior metabolic capacity to burn fat and resist toxicity. The ability to lose fat and neutralize estrogenic toxins is the key to lowering estrogen levels and to the overall success of the diet.

● ● ● **Liver detox promotes a healthy liver, creating a superior metabolic capacity to burn fat and resist toxicity.**

The most effective way to detoxify the liver is to go lower on the food chain when eating. It requires a virtual elimination of all animal food, processed grains, and wheat. The exceptions are fertile eggs and small servings of light, fresh, fermented dairy such as yogurt and kefir. Whole-grain barley, oats, and rice are allowed, as is quinoa.

Most important is the incorporation of anti-estrogenic foods and plant-derived estrogen inhibitors for the first line of defense against excess estrogen. These include, you'll remember, cruciferous vegetables, onion, garlic, citrus fruits, omega-3 oils, and wild-catch fish (optional), together with supplemental plant estrogen inhibitors, flavones, and indoles derived from passionflower, chamomile, and crucifers, respectively.

Note that natural vitamins derived from whole food sources rather than synthetic are highly bioactive, and have a superior nourishing effect on the body.

Finally, the elimination of toxins can be further enhanced via periodic fasting or undereating. The lack of food dramatically reduces the digestive stress on the body and the overall metabolic stress on the liver, thus increasing its capacity to remove toxins and utilize energy.

The Plan—Phase I

Limit food consumption to mostly raw (anti-estrogenic) fruits and vegetables or their juices, as well as small servings of light proteins, such as yogurt or fertile eggs, during the morning and early afternoon hours. That will be the best way to undereat, while maximizing liver detoxification and loading your body with anti-estrogenic nutrients. Eat your main meal in the evening. Incorporate all anti-estrogenic foods, including cruciferous vegetables, onion, garlic, and omega-3 oils, together with beans, grains, or fertile eggs. Other options for protein could be wild-catch fish or cheese.

● ◗ ● **Undereating during the day, eating mostly fresh anti-estrogenic fruits and vegetables, will greatly enhance liver detox.**

Phase I—Food List

Daytime

Oranges

Grapefruits

Berries

Broccoli sprouts

Green leafy vegetables

Celery

Carrots

Beets

Low-fat organic yogurt or kefir (8 oz.)

1–2 fertile eggs (1 yolk)

Whey protein concentrates (pesticide-free)

Also could be great as a recovery meal for athletes and other active individuals (20 g–30 g protein/serving)

Evening

Vegetables: green salad, tomatoes, onion, garlic, carrots, beets, broccoli, cauliflower, brussels sprouts, cabbage

Omega-3 oils: flaxseed, hempseed

Beans: garbanzo, pinto, black beans, etc.

Whole grains: barley, oats, rice (optional)

Sesame tahini (optional)

Protein: Fertile eggs, wild-catch fish, kefir, aged cheese

First Week—Phase I—Main Fuel

• carbohydrates

Phase I—Supplements

Estrogen Inhibitors (derived from passionflower, chamomile, and crucifers)

Milk thistle

Dandelion root

Amla C (natural vitamin C)

Shilajit (essential acids and trace minerals)

Probiotics

Multivitamins and minerals (not synthetic)

Phase I—Daily Routine Overview

Upon Waking Up

Have 1 glass of water with 5 probiotics pills, 1 magnesium pill, and 3 potassium pills. Probiotics are friendly bacteria—essential for the integral health of the digestive tract. They play a critical role in protecting the body against pathogenic bacteria such as yeast infections and digestive toxins. They also promote regularity and help relieve constipation. Elimination of waste toxins must be done on a daily basis. Bowel regularity is one of the key elements for sustaining primal health of the liver and the whole body.

● ● ●　**Regularity is one of the key elements for sustaining primal health of the liver and the whole body.**

The minerals magnesium and potassium are natural diuretics. They can help move water from the peripheral tissues to the digestive tract. Magnesium is also a great muscle relaxer and a co-factor in the synthesis of brain neurotransmitters.

From Breakfast until Lunch

A light breakfast based mostly on fruits can promote detox. Breakfast should consist of anti-estrogenic fruits such as grapefruit, oranges, or their fresh-squeezed juices. Coffee or tea is optional. Coffee is a natural diuretic and can also help to promote morning regularity. Morning supplements are multivitamins, natural vitamin C, and estrogen inhibitors.

● ● ● **The evening meal should be the biggest meal of the day.**

Active individuals including athletes, soldiers, or people engaged in intense physical training can have eggs, yogurt, or a dairy protein shake during or right after breakfast.

Those who exercise in the morning should incorporate a recovery meal made with pesticide-free whey (30 g protein) right after exercise, followed by a second, and even third, recovery meal every 1–2 hours after the initial recovery meal.

Endurance athletes can have a bowl of oatmeal or barley about one hour before training. In any case, as a general rule, the most effective way to accelerate liver detox is by incorporating the anti-estrogenic fruits on an empty stomach, every couple of hours (one fruit or one serving of berries at a time, every 2–3 hours).

From Lunch until Evening

To maintain an undereating state, lunch should also be light, but may include small servings of protein foods. Eating a green salad with a couple of poached fertile eggs can be a great lunch meal. Having yogurt and berries is another option. Dairy lovers can incorporate salad with sliced organic feta, mozzarella, or Swiss Emmental cheese (1–2 oz. per serving).

Every 2–3 hours after lunch, one can have a fruit or a protein shake. Those who work out in the afternoon should have a recovery meal after exercise.

Evening

The evening meal should be the biggest meal of the day. It should incorporate all anti-estrogenic foods, including steamed or cooked cruciferous vegetables, raw broccoli sprouts (if available), green vegetables, onion, garlic, and omega-3 oil. During the first week of liver detox, protein sources should come from combinations of beans and grains, or eggs. Other options for protein could be wild-catch fish or organic cheese (small servings). When having beans and grains such as black beans and rice, keep the ratio between beans and grain as 1:1 or 2:1. One can also incorporate beans and eggs without grains to accelerate detox and fat loss.

● ● ● **All refined sugars, soft drinks, and alcoholic beverages should be eliminated during Phase I, Liver Detox.**

The amount per serving depends upon an individual's needs and level of physical activity. Note that all refined sugars, soft drinks, and alcoholic beverages should be eliminated. Green and herbal teas are allowed and can be sweetened with 1/2 teaspoon of pure maple syrup (except for those who suffer from diabetes or blood sugar problems).

Phase I—Sample Menu

Morning: Breakfast

- 1 glass water
- 5 probiotics
- 1 grapefruit
- 1 cup coffee (freshly ground)

Mid-morning

- Organic nonfat yogurt or kefir (8 oz.) *or*
- Pesticide-free whey protein shake (30 g protein) *or*
- Cup of organic strawberries

Lunch

- Green salad and 1 teaspoon olive oil or vinaigrette (no distilled vinegar) *and*
- Two poached eggs (fertile)
- 1–2 oz. of organic cheese (optional), but carefully check how it affects you

Mid-Afternoon

- Peeled Granny Smith apple *or*
- Freshly squeezed juice—carrots, beets, parsley, celery, cucumber

Late Afternoon

- Yogurt, kefir, *or* protein shake (same as mid-morning)

Evening: Dinner

- Green salad and onions

- Steamed broccoli and garlic (2–3 large bowls),

- Black beans and rice (1:1 proportion)

- Avocado and salsa (guacamole and pico de gallo)

- 4–6 poached or boiled eggs (2 yolks), 8 oz. of wild-catch fish, or 2–3 oz. of cheese, but carefully check how it affects you

Notes

- Oats and barley can be used as an alternative to rice

- Athletes can increase amount per serving of beans, grain, and proteins

Phase I: Supplements

- Probiotics

- Multivitamins and minerals (not synthetic)

- Estrogen-inhibitor supplements

- Amla C (natural Vitamin C)

- Those who suffer from estrogen-related disorders should take increased doses of estrogen-inhibitor supplements per day

First Week Phase I Main Fuel

- Carbs from beans and grains

Best Beans

- Garbanzo (as in Hummus)
- Black
- Adzuki
- Navy

- Kidney
- White
- Great Northern
- Lentils (all kinds)

Chapter 8

Phase II: High Fat

The goal of the second week is to maximize consumption of foods that promote the anti-estrogenic hormones—progesterone in women and testosterone in men. The second week incorporates high-fat foods from the bottom of the food chain (being the second line of nutritional defense against excess estrogen). This includes raw nuts and seeds, avocado, olives, and their related oils. It also incorporates stabilized rice germ and stabilized wheat germ oils, if accessible.

During the second week, the body will be trained to shift from carbohydrate fuel to fat fuel. It is very likely, due to a superior human adaptation to primal fat fuel from raw nuts and seeds, that people may notice a slimming-down effect, in spite of the overall increase in calorie intake. The second week may also enhance virility by promoting production of anti-estrogenic sex hormones in women and men.

● ● ● **During Phase II, the body is trained to shift from carb fuel to fat fuel.**

Athletes and bodybuilders may highly benefit from the testosterone-boosting effects of raw nuts and seeds, in particular when these foods are applied in large amounts as a main fuel.

Note that the first week detox program prepares the liver for the second week by increasing its capacity to utilize fat fuel. Nevertheless, some people may react differently to a high-fat diet than others. Therefore, it is important to keep a daily progress report (i.e., energy level, body weight, performance). This data can be used later on during the following phases of the diet.

The Plan—Phase II

During the day, undereat, just as in Phase I, to maintain daily detox and enhance the liver's capacity to utilize fat and neutralize toxins. The main meal is the evening meal. Incorporate all anti-estrogenic foods as in Phase I, including greens, cruciferous vegetables, onion, garlic, and omega-3 oils. Your protein choices now also include seafood (preferably wild catch), one choice at a time. The main fuel food is raw nuts or seeds. The best nuts are almonds, pecans, and walnuts. The best seeds are pumpkin, as well as flaxseed and hemp seed (freshly ground).

Phase II—Food List

Daytime

Same as Phase I

Evening

Green salad, tomatoes, peppers, olives

Onion

Garlic

Avocado

Broccoli, cauliflower, brussels sprouts, cabbage

Omega-3 oil (flaxseed, hemp seed)

String beans

Eggplant

Eggs (preferably fertile—if not, then at least organic)

Wild-catch fish (salmon, tuna, sardines, cod, orange roughy)

Seafood (shrimp, lobster, crab)

Organic cheese

Almonds

Pecans

Walnuts

Pistachios (optional)

Pumpkin seeds

Flaxseed (freshly ground)

Hemp seed (freshly ground)

Sesame seed or tahini (optional)

Olive oil—extra virgin, cold pressed (optional)

Second Week—Phase II Main Fuel: fat.

● ◐ ● **Fat fuels consist exclusively of raw nuts and seeds.**

Note: Phase II presents a larger variety of protein choices and selection of vegetables. It also incorporates raw nuts or seeds as the main fuel-food of the meal. The most important foods in Phase II are all anti-estrogenic foods, including cruciferous vegetables, greens, onion, garlic, omega-3 oil, and, in particular, raw nuts and seeds. All other foods are important, but nevertheless, are secondary to the above list.

Phase II—Daily Routine Overview

From Wakeup until Evening

Same as Phase I

Evening

The evening meal is the main meal. It should incorporate all anti-estrogenic foods (same as Phase I) with additional choices of protein coming from seafood, preferably wild catch. The evening meal should also incorporate raw nuts and seeds as the main fuel food. Grains and bulbs (potatoes, yams, or any starchy root) should not be included.

It is recommended to adjust the amount of protein food in the meal so as to avoid feeling stuffed, and to be able to continue eating nuts or seeds towards the end of the meal without forcing oneself. As noted, athletes and other physically active individuals may increase the amount of servings per meal according to their level of activity.

Best Raw Nuts	Best Seeds
• Almonds	• Pumpkin
• Walnuts	• Flax
• Pecans	• Hemp

Raw nuts and seeds should be used as the main fuel food for the evening meal during Phase II of the diet. They should not be eaten with grains or starchy foods.

Phase II—Sample Menu

Morning—Evening

Same as Phase I

Evening

- Green salad—mixed greens, onion, pepper, and olive oil

- Sliced avocado or guacamole, and pico de gallo (diced tomatoes, onion, and lemon juice)

- Wild-catch cod cooked in tomatoes or curry sauce with cabbage, onion, and garlic; or grilled salmon marinated with olive oil and garlic; or shrimp cooked in curry sauce; organic cheese (in small amounts)

- Cooked or steamed broccoli or cauliflower

- Omega-3 oil (flaxseed or hemp seed) can be added on top of vegetables, fish, seafood, or eggs

- Raw nuts and seeds such as almonds, pecans, walnuts, pumpkin seeds, ground flaxseeds, ground hemp seeds (one choice at a time)

- Dessert—unsweetened tea

NOTES

- It is recommended to make a choice of the "protein food of the day" as well as the "nut of the day." That way, you can monitor your progress and document it according to intake of specific protein food, nuts, seeds, or combinations. This documentation will serve you later on when designing the follow-up phase.

- If you choose to use cheese, use it more as a complementary protein—not as a main source of protein in the meal

- Start with one handful of raw nuts and gradually increase the amount to see how it affects you.

Chapter 9

Phase III: Reintroduction of Foods

The goal of the third phase is to reintroduce previously restricted foods such as bread, pasta, and meats to the evening meals. The third phase is less restrictive than the previous phases, but nevertheless, it requires careful attention to how each of the reintroduced foods affects the body.

After going through the initial two phases of the diet, the body will most likely develop an increased capacity to utilize foods that may have previously caused adverse reactions (including wheat, meat, and dairy products). However, due to a high probability of an inherent intolerance to products derived from the top of the food chain, it is highly recommended to cautiously reintroduce one food at a time, carefully monitoring its effect on the body. Also, limit the reintroduction of food to no more than three times per week. Avoid soft drinks, sugar, sweets, alcoholic beverages, and low-carb products made with sugar alcohol, artificial sweeteners, or chemical preservatives.

● ● ●   **Reintroduce only one food item at a time and no more than three times in a week.**

This process requires a special attention to the following variables:

- How much of the reintroduced food was consumed per day
- How often was the reintroduced food incorporated (frequency) per week

Both the quantity of a food consumed and the frequency of food consumption could be major influences as to whether the body can tolerate a certain food or not. Therefore, the documentation of the progress must include both the quantity and the frequency of the reintroduced food, as well as how it affects the body (i.e., energy level, body weight, performance).

This progress of documenting what works and what doesn't work can help establish a most important asset—a personal database that can be used to design the follow-up phase, making the diet more viable and most effective. Note that the reintroduced food should be preferably made from organic sources and must be free of estrogenic hormones and chemicals.

The Plan—Phase III

During the day, undereat just as in the previous phases. That way, you'll be able to sustain a daily liver detox, which will help increase your body's capacity to utilize a previously restricted or problematic food.

Choose only 1–3 restricted food items at a time that you wish to bring back to the diet. Try to prioritize your food choices. Choose only food for which you really feel the need. Remember, you have only one choice at a time. For instance, if your main choice is pasta, then you won't be able to reintroduce other foods such as meats or bread at the same time.

Due to the complexity of Phase III, try keeping the right food combinations

- Do not mix carb-fuel foods with fat-fuel foods. For example, pasta and bread should not be combined with nuts or seeds, and therefore can only be incorporated with anti-estrogenic food from Phase I (i.e., detox).

- Protein, however, can be combined with both carbs and fat. Therefore, meats can combine with either nuts or grains. For that matter, meats can be incorporated with anti-estrogenic food from either Phase I or Phase II.

Reintroduce your food choice only in the main evening meal. Make sure that the other components of the diet remain the same as in previous phases.

When reintroducing food, do it for one day at a time. On the following day, go back to either detox or high fat (Phase I or Phase II, respectively). In between the intervals of reintroducing foods, try to rotate days of detox with days of high fat (Phase I–Phase II) in a manner similar to the following weekly sample:

Weekly Sample of Food Reintroduction

- Monday—meat

- Tuesday—**detox**

- Wednesday—pasta

- Thursday—high fat

- Friday—meat

- Saturday—**detox**

- Sunday—high fat

The rotation will give you a better indication of what works best for you in the long run. For instance, if you wake up the next day after reintroducing meat and feel energized and great, that's a good indication that the reintroduction of food the previous day worked well for you.

However, if you wake up and feel sluggish or nauseous or have a headache (or other untoward symptoms), this means that the reintroduction of the food the previous day did not work well. In that case, the reintroduced food should be eliminated from your diet.

Phase III—Food List
Daytime

Same as previous phases

Evening

Samples of reintroduced foods and their related combinations:

Meat or dairy combined with either Phase I (detox) foods or Phase II (high fat) foods

Bread or pasta—combine only with Phase I (detox) foods

Butter—combine with both Phase I and Phase II

Hamburger—natural hormone-free beef, no bun—combine with both Phase I and Phase II

Hamburger and buns—combine only with Phase I

Pretzels—combine only with Phase I

Cheerios—combine only with Phase I

Note

You're allowed to have only one kind of fuel food per meal.

Phase III—Daily Routine Overview

From Wake-up until Evening

Same as previous phases. Pay attention to how you feel the morning after reintroducing foods. Document your energy level and body weight. For that matter, if you exercise, make a note about your performance (i.e., strength and endurance).

Evening

This is the meal that can incorporate a previously restricted food with the right combination of anti-estrogenic food from either Phase

I or Phase II of the diet. For instance, if the reintroduced food is pasta, then the evening meal should incorporate pasta with Phase I detox foods such as greens, onion, garlic, steamed broccoli, cauliflower, or cabbage; omega-3 flaxseed oil, extra virgin olive oil, as well as eggs or fish. If the reintroduced food is meat, then the evening meal could be designed either to incorporate Phase I food, such as meat and potatoes, or instead, the evening meal can incorporate food from Phase II, such as meat and nuts.

Note

All reintroduced foods can combine with all vegetables.

Pay attention to the serving size of the reintroduced food. Start with moderate amounts such as 8 ounces of meat or a bowl of pasta, and monitor how it affects you. If everything is okay, then you can gradually increase the amount per serving of the reintroduced food, but you must carefully monitor how the increased intake affects you.

Phase III—Sample Menu

Morning—Evening

Same as previous phases

Evening—Unchanged list of foods

Green salad, onion, steamed broccoli, or cabbage with garlic, omega-3 flaxseed oil (on top of the salad), or steamed vegetables.

Reintroduced foods—samples and combinations

- Pasta—combine with the above listed food plus eggs or fish
- Bread—same as pasta
- Meat (Option 1)—Combine with the above listed foods and potatoes, beans, or grains (oat, barley, or rice)
- Meat (Option 2)—Combine with the above listed foods and raw almonds or pecans or pumpkin seeds

Phase III Main Fuel

- Carbs and fat

Chapter 10

Final Phase— The Follow Up

This final follow-up phase of the diet is built on the Phase III diet. It enables you to steadily improve your diet and take advantage of the data that you collected. This way, you'll be able to gradually establish a dietary plan that can incorporate your favorite food choices, without compromising the effectiveness of the diet.

The Plan—Final Phase

Undereat during the daily hours to promote removal of toxins from the liver and support a healthy estrogen metabolism. Take an estrogen inhibitor supplement to further enhance your defenses against excess estrogen. Your main meal should be in the evening when you can incorporate your favorite food choices, gradually evaluating how much and how often you can eat them.

To be viable, the final phase should be less restrictive so as to accommodate specific needs of different people. The following may help address various needs.

Those who wish to resume breakfast

Have light, fresh, protein foods such as poached or boiled eggs or a low-fat organic yogurt (or kefir) for your morning meal. As a general rule, a light breakfast, based on mostly fruits and tea or coffee, would help promote detox and fat burning, more than a typical full breakfast meal.

Those who wish to resume lunch

Have a clear broth or a vegetable soup, light protein such as eggs or fresh sashimi, with broccoli sprouts and a green salad. Minimize carb food consumption until the evening to avoid increased insulin resistance toward the end of the day.

Those who exercise in the morning

Have a recovery meal twenty to thirty minutes after exercise (30 g protein). It is recommended to wait twenty to thirty minutes to let the liver metabolize lactic acid. Accumulation of lactic acid after exercise is associated with a temporary state of insulin resistance. However, if the training is moderately intense or short, there is no need to wait with the recovery meal. It can be eaten right after the workout.

Those who train in the afternoon or the evening

Have a pre-exercise light meal, same as a recovery meal or half the serving size, about one hour before exercise. Eat a recovery meal after the workout as well.

Those who wish to build lean muscle mass

Incorporate 3–4 consecutive recovery meals—one every hour—after exercise. The body has an increased capacity to utilize amino acids in the muscle immediately after exercise; this anabolic capacity to utilize protein gradually diminishes within four hours. To take full advantage of the above and to finalize the actions of growth factors and growth hormone after exercise, recovery meals should be eaten within 1–4 hours after exercise. Recovery meals should be made from chemical-free, pesticide-free, fast assimilating protein, and 10–25 g of slow-releasing carbs for a swift and effective delivery of amino acids into the muscles.

Those engaged in prolonged physical activities

Those who do intense or prolonged physical activity (e.g., endurance athletes, martial artists, boxers, military, or police) should incorporate recovery meals during breaks between active periods. If the breaks are too short (e.g., 1–2 minutes), incorporate a 1/2 serving of the meal until the next break. Avoid eating full meals while under intense or prolonged physical or mental stress. That way, you'll be able to sustain a high state of alertness, while minimizing the metabolic stress on the body. Endurance athletes and other individuals engaged in prolonged physical drills can have a bowl of oatmeal or barley about one hour before training.

● ● ● **Avoid eating full meals while under intense or prolonged physical or mental stress.**

Note that all active individuals can have a handful of raw nuts or 1/2 a handful of seeds as a snack during the afternoon, instead of fruits or protein foods. Do not use trail mix, nuts, and raisins, or similar mixtures that combine nuts or seeds with high glycemic foods, in order to avoid undesirable blood sugar fluctuations and fat gain.

Those who wish to increase the amount and frequency of their favorite foods in their evening meals

Based on the data that you've already collected, if the food that you have previously reintroduced didn't cause any adverse effect, you can try to gradually increase the amount that you eat per meal, as well as the frequency that you eat this particular food per week. Do it one step at a time—start by increasing the amount per meal. Then, if that's okay, increase the frequency per week. If that's still okay, you can gradually try to increase both. That way, you can clearly evaluate how the quantity and frequency of your favorite food in your meals affect you.

● ◉ ◉ **Always stay away from estrogenic or chemically loaded food.**

With time, you'll be able to try virtually any food (except for estrogenic or chemically loaded food) in your diet, in order to learn what works for you and what does not.

Guidelines on Drinking Alcohol with Proper Food Combinations

We live in a society where regular alcohol consumption is commonplace. Many people enjoy the daily routine of having an alcoholic beverage as a means to unwind. Besides a sense of relaxation or satiation, alcohol has no real positive health effect on the body. In fact, it has just the opposite. Alcohol consumption lowers the liver's capacity to metabolize estrogen by causing ethanol toxicity, which can lead to a host of metabolic issues, including high triglycerides, insulin resistance, and high blood pressure. Therefore, alcohol, in its essence, promotes an estrogenic environment in the body. This poses the question as to whether or not one may drink and still take an anti-estrogenic approach to dieting. Quite frankly, the best action is not to drink alcohol at all. But, if you must, here are some guidelines by which you can minimize the collateral damage that alcohol may cause. All alcohol is not equal. Some choices are much worse for the body than others. What and how much you choose to drink can help to minimize or maximize any damaging effects. (Refer to the diagram at the end of this section for the best choices.)

Drink wine, preferably red, as it at least contains some nutrients that are beneficial to the body (resveratrol, tannins, anti-oxidants).

Combine alcohol only with proteins or fat-fuel foods, such as fish, eggs, nuts, or seeds, respectively (see food list from Phases I and II). Cheese is also a good combination. For that matter, wine and cheese will always be a superior combination to wine and pasta. Both the protein and fat food will help minimize an insulin spike and the negative effects on the liver.

Never eat simple or processed carbohydrate foods while drinking alcohol (e.g., crackers, cookies, pasta, grains, starches). Combining alcohol and carbs can over-spike insulin levels leading to blood sugar fluctuations, elevated blood lipids (high tryglicerides), and stubborn fat gain.

As a rule, try to incorporate as many anti-estrogenic foods as possible with alcohol. This may help balance its estrogenic effect and minimize its toxicity.

Also, stay away from drinks that are made by blending alcohol with sugary mixers (e.g., margaritas, piña coladas, fruit daiquiris, cocktails with fruit juice). These will cause a high spike in blood sugar and insulin levels.

Remember not to drink any alcohol during Phases I and II, as it would completely undermine your progress. Moreover, if you are going to drink, do so only during the Third (Reintroduction) Phase, so as to monitor how it affects your body after Liver Detoxification. Treat alcohol like a reintroduced food item. Remember, never reintroduce more than one item in the same day. This applies to alcohol as well.

If you have any existing estrogen disorders such as stubborn fat, stay away from alcohol until all of your symptoms have dissipated, so as not to prolong the issue or make it worse.

A Note about Alcohol

Having an occasional drink is not a bad thing. In fact, wine has been enjoyed for centuries in some of the greatest civilizations by people who lived long and healthy lives. Unfortunately, we now live in a world that is overwhelmed with estrogenic chemicals that already affect us in adverse ways. For those already suffering from estrogen disorders, drinking just exacerbates the issue. Therefore, it is of utmost importance to first address the estrogen issue within our bodies, so that we can effectively handle modest alcohol consumption.

Alcoholic Beverages—Best to Worst

- Red wine   BEST

- White wine

- Champagne Sec

- Vodka

- Rum

- Whisky

- Cognac

- Gin

- Sweet wines

- Sweet mixed drinks

- Liqueurs

- Beer (see Chapter 14)   WORST

The Final Phase will guide you in mastering the following skills*

- Prioritizing your food choices

- Finding your ideal fuel-food

- Incorporating anti-estrogenic foods in delicious recipes

- Incorporating traditional and ethnic dishes that can work for you

- Applying a "tactical nutrition strategy" when on the road

- Incorporating the most reliable food combinations that will never fail to keep you lean and healthy

- Utilizing the right food at the right time to enhance physical performance

*If you master these skills, you will be able to maintain your ideal body weight and prevent a weight-gain rebound while still enjoying your favorite foods.

Chapter 11

Skills Needed to Master the Diet and Never Face a Fat-Gain Rebound

Prioritizing Your Food Choices

Mastering the skill of prioritizing food choices should be your primary focus in preventing a fat-gain rebound. You'll need it every day, particularly at times when your choices of foods are limited. Your first choices should always come from the first and second lines of nutritional defense—Phase I and Phase II, respectively. Additionally, food from the bottom of the food chain will most likely work better than food from the top of the food chain. For that matter, fruits, vegetables, legumes, nuts, seeds, fertile eggs, wild-catch marine food, and organic dairy are generally superior to grains, meats, conventional dairy, and processed or chemically loaded foods. As for grains, the best choices are ancient grains including barley, oats, and rice. Quinoa, amaranth, and buckwheat are also great choices; however, they are not really grains, but rather fruits that look like grains.

Maintain the right food combinations. Your choice of fuel-food (carb or fat) should always dictate your other food choices for any particular meal. For instance, if your choice of fuel food is pasta, you can only combine it with protein foods, such as eggs or fish, but not with fat-fuel foods such as nuts and seeds.

Finally, food made with starch and sugar together, such as cookies, cakes, muffins, and commercial breads, should always be the last on the list of your food priorities. Baked goods are quite "evil" in the way they affect blood sugar, causing insulin resistance and often an undesirable fat gain. These types of foods also contribute to the problem of excess estrogen.

Finding Your Ideal Fuel Food

You can learn how the two different fuels, carb or fat, affect your body right from the start. During the final phase of the diet, you'll develop a clearer indication of what specific foods can serve you as a primary fuel. You also learn how often your primary fuel foods should be consumed per week. Finally, you will acquire the knowledge of how to cycle between carbs and fat fuels.

●   ●   ●   **Your choice of fuel food (carb or fat) should always dictate your other food choices for any particular meal.**

The skill of cycling between fuels can be used for enhancing energy utilization. Fuel cycling can help maximize glycogen-loading capacity in the muscle for explosive performance. Most importantly, when applied in a methodical manner, fuel cycling trains the body to shift from carb to fat fuel, thereby increasing its capacity to endure prolonged and intensive drills without "hitting the wall."

When determining how different fuel foods affect you, use the following parameters

- How does a specific fuel food affect your energy the day after?

- How does it affect your strength and endurance in the short and long run?

- How does it affect your weight?

Draw your conclusions after reviewing the above variables. For instance, if a specific food boosts your energy, but nevertheless causes a weight gain and a feeling of "heaviness," treat this specific food as a secondary fuel food and carefully restrict how much and how often it is consumed.

If a fuel food, however, boosts your energy while keeping you lean and "light," it can serve you as a primary fuel food and therefore can be consumed more often and in larger amounts. If any food causes adverse reactions such as allergies, headache, or fatigue, eliminate it from your diet.

Incorporating Anti-estrogenic Foods in Delicious Recipes

Make your meals tasty. Take advantage of the large variety of foods, oils, and spices listed as anti-estrogenic, and try to incorporate them into your favorite recipes. Substitute all estrogen-promoting ingredients with anti-estrogenic equivalents. For instance, if the original recipe incorporates canola or soy oil, substitute with olive oil. If an omelet is made with conventional cheese, make it instead with organic raw milk cheese—preferably uncooked—grated or sliced on top of the omelet. In the long run, the skill to create tasty meals from anti-estrogenic foods is the key to the overall viability of the diet.

 Generally, any ethnic recipe based on fresh vegetables or cooked crucifers is anti-estrogenic.

Incorporating Traditional and Ethnic Dishes That Can Work For You

Virtually all ethnic groups have traditional dishes which are anti-estrogenic. Notable among them are Mediterranean, Middle Eastern, Hispanic, and Japanese. These incorporate a large variety of vegetables, beans, fresh seafood, and fish in their recipes—all of these ingredients having anti-estrogenic properties.

Some of the dishes you can explore include Mediterranean dishes made with fresh tomatoes, vegetables, seafood, and fish, such as gazpacho or bouillabaisse; Middle Eastern dishes made with vegetables, beans, seeds, and olive oil, such as hummus, tahini, salads, and tabouli; and Hispanic dishes that use avocado, vegetables, and beans, such as guacamole, pico de gallo, and refried beans. In addition, there are grilled fish dishes popular in all the above ethnic cuisines.

Japanese sushi, pickled vegetables, and teriyaki fish are also anti-estrogenic dishes, as long as they're made without processed soy (tofu). As for soy sauce and miso soup, both are made from fermented soy and therefore contain soy isoflavones. Nonetheless, since they're typically applied in a diluted (liquid) form and in relatively small amounts (unlike tofu), it is very unlikely that they cause estrogenic effects in small servings. Saying that, just to be on the safe side, avoid cooking with miso or soy sauce to prevent a large intake of either per meal.

Many traditional and ethnic dishes counter the effects of estrogen-producing foods. Generally, any ethnic recipe based on fresh vegetables or cooked crucifers, such as cooked cabbage, is anti-estrogenic. For that matter, you can find traditional cabbage recipes in different ethnic cuisines including German, Russian, African, and Western Indian.

Appling "Tactical Nutrition Strategy" When on the Road

Millions of people these days are spending hours, days, and weeks on the road commuting, traveling, or camping. For many, being on the road is a necessity that involves prolonged periods of time spent in a car, truck, plane, or train with little or no access to fresh or unprocessed food. That includes truckers, professional drivers, military personnel, and police.

The average driver consumes whatever he or she finds in gas stations or fast food takeouts, usually eating candy bars or other junk food. This generally causes more fatigue and thus desperation for more pick-up food and so on. Consequently, truckers and other professional drivers often fail to manage their weight and sustain good health.

Military and police personnel face similar problems. Being constantly on the move or patrolling for 6–10 hours per day is highly stressful, to say the least. Due to logistical limitations, soldiers and policemen often get inadequate nutritional support, which unfortunately compromises their ability to resist fatigue and stress or to stay in shape.

● ● ● **When on the road, incorporate small meals based on low glycemic foods from the bottom of the food chain, such as fresh fruits, vegetables, light protein, raw nuts, and seeds.**

Long-distance travelers also face dietary problems. People on long flights are commonly served alcoholic beverages, fast foods, and soft drinks, which further increase the already high metabolic stress on the body. An alcoholic beverage during a flight can cause twice the damage to the liver, compared to an alcoholic beverage consumed on the ground. The body, which struggles to sustain its metabolic functions in a sealed environment at extremely high altitudes, needs to be supported by detoxifying foods rich in antioxidants as well as pure water. But instead, the overwhelmed body is hammered by alcoholic beverages, sugar-loaded soft drinks, and often heavy foods such as cold cuts and pastries. All of these have a devastating effect on the already over-stressed metabolic system, often causing inflammatory disorders, bloating, fatigue, and vulnerability to disease. To make the matter worse, all alcoholic beverages and virtually all pick-up foods are highly estrogenic, and thereby contribute to the problem of excess estrogen.

Being on the road requires a special "tactical" nutrition strategy. If you're driving, patrolling, or engaged in combat conditions, you should avoid large meals or heavy foods during the daily active hours to prevent energy crushes and constant cravings for pick-up foods. Instead, incorporate small meals based on low glycemic foods from the bottom of the food chain (listed in the first and second phases of the diet). If consumed correctly, fresh fruits, vegetables, light protein, raw nuts, and seeds can effectively nourish the body while keeping you alert, focused, and able to resist fatigue for prolonged periods of time.

To avoid not having access to these foods, pack your bag with unprocessed foods such as raw nuts or seeds. You can also use a strategy to provide yourself with a viable supply of vegetables and fruits by packing a variety of those in baby food form. Protein bars and shakes can be a great alternative for pick-up foods while on the road. Make sure they are chemical-free, low in sugar, and free of any soy.

To cover your bases, take multivitamins and minerals, as well as 1–3 doses of estrogen inhibitor supplements. Have your main meal at the end of the day or after the work is done. This is also the time to have cooked food; if you're on a night shift, eat your main meal before going to sleep.

Finally, train your body to gradually shift from carb to fat fuel. This can help you sustain steady energy levels in the long run, while keeping you lean and healthy.

Incorporating Reliable Food Combinations That Will Never Fail to Keep You Lean and Healthy

Knowing how to use food combinations that can always keep you lean and energized is the skill you need most. Even though there are differences between people's body types and food preferences, certain food combinations have been shown to work better than others in sustaining a lean physique.

● ● ● **Combinations of vegetables, beans, and eggs, such as with Phase I—Liver Detox, have proven to work wonders for fat loss in virtually all dieters.**

There is indeed a notable pattern that we have observed with our Warrior Diet followers. People who were struggling with weight fluctuations noticed that certain food combinations were always surprisingly more effective in helping them lose weight and prevent a weight-gain rebound.

The most reliable food combinations to promote fat loss were found to be those listed in the first and second lines of nutritional defense—Phases I and II of the diet, respectively.

Combinations of vegetables, beans, and eggs, such as with Phase I—Liver Detox, have proven to work wonders for fat loss in virtually all dieters. Active individuals have also reported greatly slimming down with food combinations from Phase II—High Fat. Combinations of vegetables, wild-catch fish, and raw nuts have shown to be highly beneficial not just in sustaining a lean body but also in increasing stamina and gaining strength.

In summary, food combinations from Phase I—Detox can always help you lose weight and stay lean. Food combinations from Phase II—High Fat can help you build stamina and strength while staying lean. Try to incorporate both food combinations in your weekly routine.

If you are physically active, increase the frequency of Phase II-related combinations during the week. Incorporate these high-fat food combinations in particular during workout days. Check how that works for you. If, however, your main priority is losing fat rather than just staying lean, then increase the frequency of Phase I-related combinations during the week. Check how that affects your fat loss and finally, adjust the frequencies of both food combinations according to their ongoing effects on your progress.

A SPORTS NUTRITION PROGRAM SHOULD BE BASED ON THREE CRITICAL ELEMENTS:

- Best protein food choices
- Best fuel food choices
- Best timing of meals

Utilizing the Right Food at the Right Time to Enhance Physical Performance

To effectively support a physically active lifestyle, it is of utmost importance to learn how to incorporate the right food at the right time. The skill to do that can help shorten recuperation time, promote lean muscular development, and improve performance.

A sports nutrition program should be based on three critical elements: best protein food choices, best fuel food choices, and best timing of meals. Physically active individuals require a higher food intake than sedentary people. For that matter, food must be carefully selected to avoid undesirable fat gain and other metabolic disorders. It must be free of chemicals and estrogenic substances.

Best protein food choices

A GOOD PROTEIN SOURCE SHOULD HAVE
THE FOLLOWING PROPERTIES:

- Provide all essential amino acids in the right ratio
  (complete protein)
- Easily digested and fast-assimilated
- Fresh, minimally processed, and chemical free

Today, many protein foods and products are over-processed, loaded with chemicals, or past their expiration date, all of which render them unfit for human consumption. Over-processing—such as creating isolated proteins—often involves massive chemical reactions with acid detergents and high temperatures that destroy sensitive essential amino acids (such as methionine and lysine), leading to formation of deficient proteins.

To avoid that, choose protein foods that are fresh and minimally processed. Your best bets are organic dairy products, organic eggs (preferably fertile), and wild-catch fish.

Dairy proteins from fresh milk products or whey are assimilated relatively quickly, and provide all essential amino acids and immuno-supporting globulins. Combining whey and milk proteins together can help support immediate recuperation and long-lasting muscle nourishment.

Best Choices of Fuel Foods

(FOODS TO GIVE YOUR BODY ENERGY)

CARBOHYDRATES: FATS:

- Whole Barley   - Raw Almonds

- Steel-cut Oats   - Walnuts

- Whole-grain rice   - Pecans

- Quinoa

- Amaranth

Eggs are another great protein choice. They provide all essential amino acids, and in particular, the amino acids methionine and lysine, which are often destroyed in protein foods due to cooking or over-processing. The yolk in eggs provides critical nutrients including DNA, RNA, vitamins, amino acids, N-3, and lecithin. The yolk contributes to the high biological value of eggs' protein. Do not eat egg whites alone. Always combine the white with the yolk in ratios between 1–4 whites to 1 yolk. Choose fertile eggs if possible. Distinct from conventional infertile eggs, fertile eggs generally have a superior nutritional composition.

Wild-catch fish is also a great source of protein. Fish is easier to digest than meat. It is also a great source of omega-3 oils in their most bioactive form. Compared to meat and poultry, fish is a superior protein food with profound anti-inflammatory and immuno-supportive properties.

The human body has primarily adapted to utilize only two kinds of fuels: carbs and fat. Our bodies are not efficient in utilizing protein as a primary fuel. Unlike other predators, we lack enzymes that convert degraded D proteins into live L proteins and thus, through evolution, we have become limited in our capacity to consume animal meat (if it wasn't fresh-kill, cured, or cooked, it couldn't fit human consumption). Using protein as a fuel involves a substantial waste of nitrogen with consequential increased levels of nitrites and nitrates, all of which adversely affect the circulatory and muscular systems.

● ● ● **Note that all living organisms on this planet are made from L proteins (L stands for *levo* or left). Yet, upon death of an organism, L proteins convert into mirror-image D proteins (D stands for *devo*). This spontaneous conversion of live L protein into dead (or raceant) D proteins is a process that typically occurs during rotting of meat. The human body has no capacity to protect itself from D proteins. Indeed, accumulation of D protein in the tissues was found to be associated with accelerated aging and diseases such as Parkinsons and Alzheimers.**

Unlike protein, both carbs and fat can be incorporated as a fuel food. Nevertheless, one should use either carbs or fat according to one's needs.

The best choices for carb fuel are the lower glycemic ancient grains—whole barley, oats, and rice. Quinoa and amaranth are also good, but often aren't as easily accessible. Carbs are quickly assimilated and therefore can support an immediate recovery. Carb-fuel foods can be also used for glycogen loading before intense or prolonged physical activity. Body-builders can take advantage of carb fuel to induce insulin activity and thus enhance the overall anabolic effect of meals after exercise.

Long before the appearance of carb-fuel foods, humans had already adapted to survive on fat-fuel foods. Unlike carbs, fat fuel is slow releasing and works for a longer lasting period of time. Your best choices of fat-fuel foods are raw nuts such as almonds, walnuts, and pecans. Raw almonds are alkalizing and easier to digest than other nuts. Use fat-fuel foods to increase your stamina and stay lean through your lifetime. Training your body to gradually shift from carb to fat fuel is a long-term investment in your future capacity to generate energy and sustain a lean physique. Fat-fuel foods would be a better choice for the purpose of sheer fat loss, by virtue of their low-glycemic and slow-releasing effect on the body.

You have a 3–4 hour window after a workout to incorporate recovery meals effectively.

THEY SHOULD BE PLANNED AS FOLLOWS:

1st hour	20–30 g protein
	10–25 g carbs.
2nd hour	20–30 g protein
3rd hour	20–30 g protein
4th hour	20–30 g protein

Best Timing of Meals

The most critical meals for an individual doing physical training are post-exercise recovery meals. After exercise, the body is in a peak anabolic potential with a substantial increased capacity to utilize protein and other nutrients in the muscle tissue. This window of opportunity diminishes gradually within 3–4 hours after exercise. To take advantage of this post-exercise period, incorporate recovery meals based on fresh, light, and fast-releasing proteins such as whey and milk (20 g–30 g) together with low-glycemic carbs (10–25 g per meal). That way you'll be able to nourish the muscle with amino acids and carb fuel for immediate recuperation, glycogen loading, and to also promote a lean muscle-mass gain. You can incorporate 2–3 consequential recovery meals after an intense drill, every 1–2 hours.

Your main evening meal can incorporate slow-releasing foods such as cooked fish, an omelet, or raw nuts. That can help facilitate long-lasting nutrient release during the night for a profound recuperation, buildup of tissues, and final reloading of energy reserves for the next day.

Note: Minimize your consumption of cooked slow-releasing foods during the day. They may cause an increase in digestive stress and slow you down during your active hours. Also, due to their slow-releasing effect, they can't be adequately used for fast recovery after exercise. However, slow-releasing raw foods such as sashimi, nuts, and seeds can be used as small snacks during the day, except for post-exercise recovery.

Chapter 12

How the Anti-Estrogenic Diet Can Help Address Different Disorders

Those Who Suffer from Adverse Reactions to Certain Foods

If you suffer from adverse reactions to certain foods—whether in the form of allergies, headaches, fatigue, bloating, weight gain, or irritability—you may have an existing intolerance to a certain food. Check your database. Eliminate the last reintroduced food for a few days. Check if the increase in the amount per meal or the frequency per week is the reason for your reactions. Adjust the amount or frequency accordingly. If that doesn't help and the reaction reoccurs, eliminate this food from your diet. If you suffer from a reaction to a food that was just reintroduced, avoid eating this food.

After the elimination of a problematic food, incorporate 1–3 days of detox (Phase I) and then resume eating meals with your favorite foods. It is important though to keep detox days as well as high fat days in your weekly routine. Some individuals may realize that one detox day per week is sufficient enough, while others may realize that they require more.

Some people, in particular those who are physically active, may find that training their bodies to gradually shift into fat fuel (Phase II) can help increase their stamina and overall capacity to endure an intense and prolonged stress—and all that while thinning down.

Those Who Suffer from Estrogen-Related Disorders

Stubborn fat

Stubborn fat is estrogen-sensitive fatty tissue that is highly responsive to estrogen activity. When in excess, estrogen promotes the growth of estrogen-sensitive fatty tissues, particularly in the belly and waist, as well as other estrogen-sensitive areas such as: the chest in men; the lower buttocks, upper thighs, and back of the arms in women.

● ● ●   **Be patient! The elimination of stubborn fat requires time and work.**

Estrogen-sensitive fatty tissue generally resists fat-burning because of its high affinity to estrogen, which is a fat-gain-promoting hormone. Furthermore, estrogen-sensitive tissues, belly fat in particular, are also the site for estrogen synthesis via an enzymatic process called aromatizing. This process is responsible for the conversion of androgens to estrogen in both sexes. This causes a vicious cycle of fat gain in which excess estrogen promotes fat gain and the enlarged fatty tissue produces even more estrogen that further accelerates fat gain, and so forth.

To effectively get rid of stubborn fat, start by eliminating all estrogen-promoting foods and chemicals from your diet. That includes all soy products, omega-6-rich oils (such as corn, canola, safflower, rapeseed, and soy), animal-fat rich foods, conventional meats and dairy, low-carb and weight-loss products containing petroleum-based synthetic ingredients such as sugar alcohol, artificial sweeteners, glycerin, and chemical preservatives. Avoid white sugar, fructose, candies, soft drinks, and alcoholic beverages.

To jump-start the diet, incorporate 1–3 weeks of detox (Phase I) together with a steady exercise routine. Take 2–3 servings of estrogen inhibitors every day. Try to exercise on an empty stomach or while undereating to maximize the slimming down and estrogen-lowering effects of your workout.

Check how detox affects your progress. Move into Phase II and Phase III of the diet, and keep documenting how different fuels and foods affect your progress. Over time, you'll know what foods work for you and what do not. Nonetheless, in times of setbacks or confusion, switch back to detox, or simply incorporate food mostly from the bottom of the food chain. This trick always works. Be patient. The elimination of stubborn fat requires time and work. Nevertheless, by being persistent you'll be able to notice a substantial slimming-down effect in areas of your body that were previously totally resistant to fat burning.

Note that your body-fat percentage is regulated by a certain innate mechanism that dictates optimum set levels of body fat. You can take advantage of this mechanism and gradually lower your body-fat percentage set-point. Studies have revealed that certain proteins called AMP kinase, which are copiously produced during fasting, undereating, and exercise, are responsible for giving the body the signal to lower its body-fat set-point. Therefore, the incorporation of undereating or fasting, together with exercise, is the most effective method to break a fat-loss plateau and also reset a lower optimum body-fat percentage, thereby preventing a fat-gain rebound.

⬤ ◐ ⬤ **In times of setbacks or confusion, switch back to Phase I Detox.**

Combining the Anti-Estrogenic Diet and supplements with an effective exercise routine most likely will give the best results in losing weight and staying lean while developing high resilience to stress and disease.

PMS

The main culprit for PMS, it is now known, is excess estrogen. If you suffer from PMS symptoms (i.e., heavy bleeding, bloating, cramps, and fatigue), start by incorporating 1–3 weeks of detox (Phase I), while taking 2–3 servings daily of estrogen inhibitors. Some women may feel a relief immediately; others may notice a substantial alleviation of PMS symptoms only in the second menstrual cycle after starting the diet. When symptoms subside, add high fat (Phase II) days to your weekly schedule to promote production of the anti-estrogenic hormone progesterone. When you reach the final phase of the diet, make sure that your food choices are safe. Nonetheless, try to incorporate 1–3 days of detox per week. You may also find that gradually increasing consumption of raw nuts and seeds as a main fuel food can be highly beneficial. Check how changes in the diet affect your energy level and body weight. In case of a setback, resume detox and remove problematic food from your diet.

Endometriosis and Fibrocystic disease

Same routine as PMS. Application of progesterone cream could be highly beneficial. Check with your physician. Also, maximize consumption of cruciferous vegetables and omega-3 oil. Take 2–3 daily servings of estrogen inhibitors.

Women on HRT

Same routine as PMS. Take 2–3 servings of estrogen inhibitors as an extra protection against excess estrogen. Women who are under hormonal replacement therapy (HRT) may suffer from excess estrogen due to a low level of progesterone. To address that, you can use progesterone cream after consulting with your physician. If you're taking pure estrogen drugs, you may be in the highest risk margin. If this is the case, get a second opinion. Do your own research about HRT and find a physician who can help you incorporate balanced HRT (estrogen and progesterone) instead of pure estrogen.

Women who suffer from premenopausal symptoms

Same routine as PMS. Premenopausal women suffer from a substantial loss of progesterone. Try to incorporate 2–3 days of high fat (Phase II) per week in the final phase. If that helps, increase the number of high fat days per week and check if that works for you. Try applying progesterone cream, after consulting with your physician. Check how that affects your symptoms.

Menopausal women

Same as for premenopausal women. You might consider HRT. Do your research. Do not take unbalanced HRT estrogen drugs (i.e., estrogen alone without progesterone) to avoid excess of estrogen in the body and related increased risk for cancer. Find a physician who can help you.

Men who suffer from prostate enlargement

There is evidence that excess estrogen contributes to growth of the prostate gland. A direct correlation was also found between harmful estrogen metabolites (16 alpha-hydroxy estrogens) and prostate enlargement. To defend your body against prostate enlargement and its related symptoms, incorporate 1–3 weeks of detox (Phase I) and take 2–3 daily servings of estrogen-inhibitor supplements. Check your PSA before and after incorporating detox. If the PSA level goes down, move into Phase II of the diet and keep supplementing 2–3 daily servings of estrogen inhibitors. Be very careful with your food choices during Phase III of the diet; certain foods such as meats and conventional milk products may cause setbacks. A vegetarian diet (with no soy) could be a highly beneficial alternative in cases of prostate enlargement. Finally, exercise at least three times per week. Exercise is associated with a lower risk for prostate-related disorders and cancer

● ◉ ●   **Meats and conventional milk products may cause setbacks for those with prostate problems.**

Type II Diabetes

The Anti-Estrogenic Diet can help eliminate estrogen-sensitive belly fat and reduce waist size, lowering the risk for developing insulin-resistant diabetes.

Type II diabetes is a clinical state of insulin resistance, involving chronic elevation of blood-sugar levels, high levels of blood lipids, and often a condition called "fatty liver." In a late stage, diabetes can lead to neural degradation and an overall metabolic decline. Diabetes is often associated with being overweight, obesity, and hypertension (Syndrome X). Treatments generally involve the use of drugs.

● ● ● **People who are hypoglycemic, hyperglycemic, or have Type II diabetes can surprisingly reverse their condition without the use of drugs.**

However, independent studies reveal that drugs aren't the only solution. People who are hypoglycemic, hyperglycemic, or have Type II diabetes can reverse their condition without the use of drugs. There is a growing amount of evidence that simple methods such as liver detox, exercise, and consumption of low glycemic meals can effectively help reestablish insulin sensitivity and healthy levels of blood sugar.

Liver detoxification is critically important. When the liver is overwhelmed by chemicals, drugs, alcohol, or lipids, it gradually loses its ability to metabolize fat. This causes an accumulation of fat metabolites in the liver (fatty liver). Under this condition, the liver fails to utilize glucose, creating a state of insulin resistance.

To reverse this, incorporate 1–3 weeks of liver detox (Phase I), and take 1–2 servings of estrogen inhibitors per day to protect your liver and your body from estrogenic chemicals. If possible try to exercise at least three times per week. When applying detox, try to substitute grains with beans, or keep a high ratio, 2:1, of beans to grains. Check how this regimen affects your blood sugar. If your blood sugar drops to below 100, gradually incorporate days of high fat (Phase II) into your weekly schedule.

If the blood sugar drops further, it's a sign that you can gradually eliminate the drugs (if you take any). Consult with your physician.

While establishing a healthy level of blood sugar, try to eat only low glycemic meals, while training your body to shift from carb fuel to the lower glycemic fat fuel found in raw nuts and seeds. Keep a steady exercise routine with a high frequency of workouts per week. Also, train while undereating to maximize the beneficial effects of exercise on slimming down, lowering blood sugar levels, and stabilizing insulin.

Note that insulin resistance is often associated with central obesity—i.e., excess belly fat (a "pear shape")—which is also associated with excess estrogen.

Hypertension

Hypertension involves high blood pressure, high blood lipids, salt sensitivity, and often insulin resistance, all of which are called Syndrome X. Researchers found that Syndrome X is typically associated with a large waist size (belly fat) which gives the body a "pear shape." Excessive belly fat is also associated with excess estrogen.

To reverse the problem, hypertensive people should try to lose weight, particularly in the belly area. To effectively treat hypertension, one should incorporate a steady workout routine.

The Anti-Estrogenic Diet can be most beneficial in this case by helping eliminate stubborn belly fat, counteracting excess estrogen, and removing toxins from the liver. That will help create the right metabolic environment for lowering cholesterol and blood lipid levels, while normalizing blood pressure. If you suffer from hypertension-related symptoms, incorporate a similar plan as was addressed previously with diabetes (see type II diabetes).

● ● ● **By detoxifying the liver, lowering blood lipids, lowering blood pressure, and losing weight, you may be able to reverse your condition and sustain a healthy body.**

Note that in case of hypertension, whole grains such as oats and barley could be highly beneficial. The fiber in these grains is rich in some of the most potent cholesterol-lowering compounds, called proteoglucans. Incorporate oats or barley during the detox phase. If that works well, you can have these grains as your main fuel food. However, if you suffer from insulin resistance (hypoglycemia), follow the same program as with Type II diabetes, gradually training your body to use raw nuts and seeds as your main fuel food.

Cardiovascular Disorders

Cardiovascular disorders are associated with symptoms that are similar to hypertension and insulin resistance. There is indeed a direct correlation between high cholesterol, high triglycerides, high blood pressure, high blood sugar, and a high risk for cardiovascular disease, as well as heart attack. To address the problem, follow the same plan as previously addressed with hypertension. By detoxifying the liver, lowering blood lipids, lowering blood pressure, and losing weight, you may be able to reverse your condition and sustain a healthy body. If you take blood pressure or cholesterol-lowering drugs, consult with your physician before discontinuing use.

Digestive Disorders

Digestive disorders such as indigestion, heartburn, esophageal disorders, and food intolerance are often caused by underlying metabolic problems including a lack of enzymes, intolerance to foods, chemical toxicity, and chronic constipation. One of the major contributors to the problem is eating too frequently. Eating meals too often may not allow the body enough time to recuperate between meals and reload its enzyme pool. This can cause a lack of enzymes and hydrochloric acid in the stomach, leading to the development of digestive disorders with conditions such as acid reflux (heartburn), esophageal disorders, and food intolerance.

The loss of enzymes and hydrochloric acid causes a condition called an "alkaline stomach." When the stomach lacks an optimum level of pH, protein digestion is severely compromised, leading to an inadequate utilization of amino acids. This further accelerates the loss of enzymes and, thus, overall digestive power.

● ● ● **A major contributor to digestive disorders is eating too frequently.**

Digestive disorders can cause a vicious cycle where the body is exposed to an ever-growing level of undigested food particles along with metabolic waste, all of which increase the metabolic stress on the liver. Thus, the overwhelmed liver loses its capacity to neutralize harmful toxins including estrogenic chemicals. The loss of digestive power leaves the body vulnerable to chemical toxicity and the harmful effects of excess estrogen.

To treat digestive disorders, jump-start the diet by incorporating intensive 1–3 weeks of liver detox. Supplement this with liver detoxifying herbs, 1–3 servings of estrogen inhibitors, and additional 2–3 caps of probiotics daily before sleep.

If you find through testing that you suffer from alkaline stomach, take HCL and/or enzyme supplements 20–30 minutes before your main meal. Consult with your physician. Eating papaya or pineapple during the day can be highly beneficial. Both fruits are rich in protease enzymes which are also known for their anti-inflammatory properties.

If you suffer from over-acid stomach, incorporate 1–3 weeks of liver detox. However in this case, try applying only alkaline-forming foods in your meals. Examples of alkaline-forming foods are fruits, vegetables, raw almonds, salt, and chamomile tea. To avoid an acid reaction, do not eat sour fruits until symptoms subside. Also, avoid all acid-forming foods such as onion, garlic, meat, all wheat products (including pasta), roasted nuts, fried or seared food, and ice water. Rice and quinoa may work well as they are not acid-forming grains. Finally, supplement with all essential nutrients, vitamins, and minerals—in particular, calcium (at least 1–2 g a day).

When symptoms subside, move gradually to the final phase, carefully checking how each of your favorite (reintroduced) foods affects you. Do not take any unnecessary risks. If some foods cause reactions, eliminate them from your diet.

● ● ● **If untreated, irregularity can lead to severe metabolic disorders as well as cancer.**

To regain digestive power, try to eat one main meal per day. During the day, consume mostly alkalizing foods such as raw fruits and vegetables. You can also have light, fresh, protein foods (preferably organic). Have cooked and acid-forming foods such as grains, fish, or meat in your evening meal. That way, you'll be able to maintain a balanced diet, nourishing your body with fresh detoxifying food during the daily hours, while giving it the time to recuperate and reestablish its digestive power toward the evening. Note that the whole cycle of eating-digesting-recuperating is critically important. If one of the cycle's links is compromised, disorders and disease will most likely reoccur.

Irregularity

Being "irregular" ironically is very a "regular" occurrence in this country. Laxative drugs are sold over-the-counter as commonly as pain-relief medications. Unfortunately, drugs do not treat the core of the problem. If anything, they make it worse. If untreated, irregularity can lead to severe metabolic disorders as well as cancer.

● ● ● **The most notable cause of irregularity is a deficiency in friendly gut bacteria.**

The inability to regulate a healthy daily cycle of elimination causes an accumulation of waste toxins and a reverse flash of "dirty" bile acids from the guts to the liver. Bile acids are made from liver cholesterol and play a critical role in the metabolism of dietary fat. After digestion, bile acids, attached to waste toxins, should normally be eliminated out of the body. However, when constipation occurs, the bile-waste complex is instead mobilized back to the liver. The overwhelmed liver is now forced to detoxify, neutralize, and metabolize the toxic-bile complex as well as its related cholesterol. This continuous onslaught of toxins weakens the liver and lowers its capacity to metabolize fat and glucose. Consequently, this can lead to elevation of blood lipids, elevation of blood pressure, and fluctuation of blood sugar with symptoms that include allergies, headache, irritability, bloating, and weight gain.

Irregularity has various causes, including low intake of dietary fiber and a high intake of processed foods. Nonetheless, the most notable cause is a deficiency in "friendly" gut bacteria, also known as "probiotics." Ideally, probiotics should colonize the digestive tract in a ratio of more than 10 times higher than pathogenic bacteria. Unfortunately, it is most common today to find the opposite. When there is a surplus of pathogenic bacteria rather than friendly bacteria in the digestive tract, individuals may suffer from yeast infections and related symptoms including allergies, fatigue, and chronic constipation.

To treat irregularity, follow the same program as previously addressed with the above digestive disorders. Adjust the amount of daily probiotics supplements and potassium supplements according to your needs. You may require a larger amount of daily probiotics supplements to fight an existing infection and reverse your condition. Also, you may need to incorporate 2–3 days of liver detox per week during the final phase of the diet. That way, you'll provide your digestive system and your liver with the means to recuperate and sustain healthy functions in the long run.

Chapter 13

Recipes

The following recipes target different phases of the diet and can help you jump-start the diet as well as serve as tasty dishes for the follow-up phase. Hopefully, this will help you enjoy the diet, while becoming leaner and healthier. The previous chapters show how to make proper food choices. Be creative, try various anti-estrogenic food combinations, and adjust recipes according to your personal taste. Feel free to submit your recipes to us via our forum on www.DefenseNutrition.com. We'll update the website with these recipes as we receive them.

Note that for Phase II, raw unsalted nuts or seeds will be eaten after meals.

● Hummus
(Phases I, II, and III)

2 cups canned garbanzo beans (drained)

1/3 cup tahini

1/4 cup lemon juice

1 teaspoon sea salt

2 cloves garlic, halved

1 tablespoon olive oil

1 pinch paprika

1 teaspoon fresh parsley, minced

Directions

1. Place the garbanzo beans, tahini, lemon juice, salt, and garlic in a blender or food processor. Blend until smooth.

2. Transfer mixture to a serving bowl.

3. Drizzle olive oil over the garbanzo bean mixture. Sprinkle with paprika and parsley.

● Black Bean Hummus
(Phases I, II, and III)

3 cloves garlic

3 (15-oz.) cans black beans

1/4 cup lemon juice

5 tablespoons sesame tahini

2 tablespoons ground cumin

1 tablespoon ground cinnamon

1 teaspoon salt (sea salt)

1/2 teaspoon cayenne pepper

1/2 teaspoon paprika

Directions

1. Mix all ingredients in a blender or food processor until smooth.

2. Serve with vegetables.

● Robin's Spicy Black Bean Soup
(Phases I, II, and III)

1 tablespoon extra-virgin olive oil

1/2 large red onion, chopped

2 tablespoons minced garlic

1 (14.5-oz.) can diced tomatoes with green chili peppers

1 head cabbage, chopped

1/4 cup fresh cilantro, chopped

1 teaspoon cayenne pepper

1 cup fresh tomatoes, chopped

1 dash chili powder

1 dash cumin

1 dash ground cinnamon

2 (15-oz.) cans black beans (drained)

3 cups organic low-sodium chicken broth

Directions

1. Heat oil in a saucepan over medium heat.

2. Stir in onion and cook about 2 minutes; then stir in garlic and cook until onion is soft and translucent.

3. Stir in tomatoes, cabbage, cilantro, and chicken broth. Season with cayenne pepper, chili powder, cumin, and ground cinnamon. Cook for 10 minutes.

4. Stir in black beans and bring to a simmer. Reduce to low heat, cover and simmer 1 hour or longer.

● Simple Lentil Soup
(Phases I, II, and III)

1 pound dried lentils

2 garlic cloves, chopped

2 celery stalks, chopped

1 medium onion, chopped

Salt and pepper to taste

8 cups water

Directions

1. Combine above ingredients and water in soup pot.

2. Bring to boil then reduce heat to medium and simmer for 30–45 minutes. Lentils will be tender when done.

● Ann's Bean Soup
(Phases I, II, and III)

1 cup red kidney beans

1 cup white kidney beans

1 cup black or navy beans

1 cup chick peas

1 bay leaf

2 tablespoons thyme

1 tablespoon turmeric

1/2 red cabbage

2 red onions

1 red bell pepper

1 yellow bell pepper

1 orange bell pepper

1 green bell pepper

3 stalks celery

2 medium yellow squash

2 medium zucchini

1 large can tomatoes

1 small can tomatoes

Directions

1. Soak all dried beans together overnight in large pot. Rinse several times before cooking.

2. Cook beans on medium high in water in large pot for 1 hour with bay leaf and turmeric.

3. Chop all vegetables and add to soup pot along with 2 tablespoons thyme.

4. Cook soup on medium, adding more water as needed until ingredients cook down. This should take about 30–40 minutes.

5. This makes a large pot, so be prepared to freeze what you don't use.

● Black Lentil Soup
(Phases I, II, and III)

2 cups dried black lentils

1 stalk celery

1 large carrot

1 large onion

5–6 cloves garlic

2 teaspoons cumin

4 cups hot water

Salt and pepper to taste

Directions

1. Pour 2 cups of the hot water over the dried lentils; leave the rest to the side.

2. Cut the celery, carrot, and onion into a small dice. Mince garlic. Combine all ingredients in a large stock pot. Saute until the onion and celery are translucent (be careful not to burn the garlic).

3. Drain the lentils. Add the lentils and cumin and stir. Add the remaining 2 cups of water and bring to a boil.

4. Reduce heat to a light simmer for 45 minutes or until lentils are tender.

5. Salt and pepper to taste.

● Black Bean & Salsa Soup (Phases I, II, and III)

2 (15-oz.) cans black beans, drained and rinsed

1-1/2 cups vegetable broth

1 cup chunky salsa

1 teaspoon ground cumin

4 tablespoons organic sour cream

2 tablespoons green onion, thinly sliced

Directions

1. In electric food processor or blender, combine beans, broth, salsa, and cumin. Blend until fairly smooth.

2. Heat the bean mixture in a medium-sized saucepan over medium heat until thoroughly heated. To serve, ladle soup into 4 individual bowls and top each bowl with 1 tablespoon of the sour cream and 1/2 teaspoon green onion.

● Oatmeal and Eggs (Phase III)

2–3 cups oatmeal (rolled oats or steel-cut oats)

6–12 egg whites with 2–4 yolks

1/4 teaspoon turmeric (optional)

1/4 teaspoon cumin (optional)

Salt and pepper to taste

1/2 cup cilantro, coarsely chopped for garnish

Directions

1. Fill a large pot with 4–5 cups water and bring to a boil. Add oatmeal and spices. Rolled oats need half the time that steel-cut oats need (check the preparation instructions on the box). If you choose steel-cut oats, soak them overnight in purified, steam-distilled, or spring water to cut down on cooking time

2. Reduce heat and let cook until almost done. Stir occasionally to avoid clumping.

3. When you notice that very little water is left, add the eggs and slowly mix it all together.

4. Once the eggs are thickening, turn the stove off, cover pot, and let it simmer for a couple of minutes.

5. Garnish with cilantro and serve.

This high-carbohydrate meal goes very well with buttermilk or kefir for additional protein and beneficial bacteria. The buttermilk and kefir can be used as a cooling sauce you put on top. This dish also goes well with steamed broccoli and cauliflower.

If you'd like to make this dish spicier, you can add curry or cumin. It can also be garnished with scallions or chopped onions. Use your imagination. With trial and error, you'll find what's best for you.

● Egg Omelet with Tomato Sauce
(Phases I, II, and III)

16 egg whites with 3–4 yolks

1/4 cup of tomato sauce or crushed tomatoes

1/4 small onion, diced (optional)

1 tablespoon olive oil

Salt and cayenne pepper to taste

Parsley or cilantro, chopped

Directions

1. Preheat olive oil in a large, deep skillet. Add diced onions and sear until browned.

2. Slowly add tomato sauce, mix with onions.

3. When sauce is boiling, add the eggs. Scramble and mix the eggs while cooking.

4. When mixture thickens, remove from the stove, put in a large bowl and cover.

5. Serve garnished with the chopped parsley or cilantro.

Those who like mushrooms can steam or sauté in olive oil shiitake or portabella mushrooms for use as a topping. Or, they can be cooked with the omelet.

Egg omelets go very well with steamed zucchini, butternut squash, steamed pumpkin, sweet peas, and black bean soup, which you can also use as a topping.

● Omelet with Black Beans
(Phases I, II, and III)

This uses the same preparation as the above omelet, only in this case, you use black bean soup instead of tomato sauce. You can use a half-can of organic black bean soup, available in most health-food stores and supermarkets.

● Scrambled Egg Delight
(Phases I, II, and III)

5 whole fertile eggs

5 egg whites from fertile eggs

1 green bell pepper

1 red bell pepper

1 yellow bell pepper

1 white onion

1 large tomato

1 clove garlic

2 tablespoons olive oil

Directions

1. Chop all vegetables. Heat large skillet adding olive oil, then vegetables.

2. Sauté for 5 minutes.

3. Add eggs and scramble together until eggs are cooked.

● Lentil Quiche
(Phases I, II, and III)

1 cup onion, chopped

2 tablespoons olive oil

1/2 cup dried lentils

1 cups water

1 cup organic chicken broth

2 cups broccoli florets

1 cup fresh tomatoes, chopped

4 eggs, beaten

1 cup organic milk (raw milk is best)

1 teaspoon sea salt

Dash of cayenne pepper (optional)

1/2 cup organic mozzarella cheese, shredded (optional)

Directions

1. Preheat oven to 375°. Place onion and olive oil into a 9-inch deep-dish pie plate. Bake for about 15 minutes, or until onion is tender.

2. Place the lentils and water into a saucepan and bring to a boil. Cook for about 20 minutes, or until lentils are tender. Drain most of the water off, then place the broccoli florets on top of the lentils. Cover and cook for about 5 minutes. This will dry the lentils and cook the broccoli.

3. Transfer the lentils, broccoli, and tomatoes to the pie plate with the onions, and stir to evenly distribute each item. Stir in

cheese at this time if using. In a medium bowl, whisk together the eggs, milk, chicken broth, sea salt, and cayenne pepper. Pour over the ingredients in the pie plate.

4. Bake for 45 minutes in the preheated oven, or until the center is firm when the quiche is jiggled. Cool for a few minutes before slicing and serving.

● Oatmeal Pancakes
(Phase III)

1/2 cup oats

1/4 cup low-fat organic cottage cheese

2 eggs

1 teaspoon vanilla extract

1/4 teaspoon cinnamon

1/4 teaspoon nutmeg

1 tablespoon butter

Directions

1. Process the oatmeal, cottage cheese, eggs, vanilla extract, cinnamon, and nutmeg in a blender until smooth.

2. Melt the butter in a frying pan. Add the batter and cook over medium heat until bubbles appear, then flip and cook other side, until both sides are lightly browned.

● Guacamole Dip
(Phases I, II, and III)

2 very ripe avocados

2 tablespoons onion, chopped fine

1 clove garlic, minced

1/2 red bell pepper, cut fine

1/2 green bell pepper, cut fine

1 medium ripe tomato, peeled and chopped

2 stalks celery, chopped fine

1 tablespoon lime or lemon juice

Directions

1. Halve the avocados, remove pits, and scoop flesh into a glass container.
2. Mash with a fork and blend in remaining ingredients. Serve as quickly as possible.
3. Serve with fresh vegetables.

● High Essential Fat Salad
(Phases I, II, and III)

Organic mixed herbs or greens

1/4 organic avocado, sliced

1 artichoke heart (cut up)

5 pitted kalamata olives

5 organic grape tomatoes

1 teaspoon organic flax or hemp seeds, ground

1 tablespoon olive or flax seed oil

1 tablespoon organic apple cider vinegar

Directions

1. Using above ingredients, prepare each salad serving on its own plate.

2. Place mixed herbs or greens on plate. Next, place artichoke and avocado on top of greens.

3. Place 5 kalamata olives and 5 tomatoes on top for presentation.

4. Sprinkle a teaspoon of flax or hemp seed on top and then add oil and vinegar.

5. Keep in mind that since this salad is high in good fat, it is quite filling. You may want make two portions of it.

● Coconut Shrimp and Vegetables
(Phases II and III)

1 head cauliflower

1 cup okra

1 cup cannellini (white) beans

1 onion, chopped

1 cup of shiitake mushrooms

1 pound shrimp, peeled

1/2 cup organic coconut milk

1 cup organic vegetable broth

1 tablespoon organic unsalted butter

1 tablespoon soy sauce

Directions

1. Combine all ingredients, except for shrimp.

2. Simmer for 20 minutes with lid on, stirring occasionally.

3. When 5 minutes is left on timer, add shrimp.

● Spinach-Stuffed Flounder with Mushrooms and Feta (Phases II and III)

8 large fresh mushrooms, sliced

8 oz. spinach, rinsed and chopped

1 tablespoon feta cheese, crumbled

4 (4-oz.) flounder fillets

Directions

1. Preheat oven to 350°.

2. Wipe medium-sized skillet with olive oil. Heat over medium heat. Add the mushrooms and cook about 5 minutes or until the liquid released from the mushrooms has evaporated, stirring occasionally.

3. Add the spinach to the skillet. Cook and stir about 2 minutes or until spinach is wilted. Remove from the heat and drain excess moisture. Sprinkle the feta cheese over the vegetables, then stir.

4. To assemble the fish rolls, place one-quarter of the spinach mixture onto the wide end of each filet. Carefully roll the filet around the spinach mixture. Use wooden toothpicks to hold the end of each roll in place.

5. Wipe an 8 x 8-inch baking dish with olive oil. Place the fish rolls, seam side down, in the baking dish. Add 2 tablespoons of water. Loosely cover with foil.

6. Bake in a preheated oven for 15–20 minutes or until fish flakes easily when tested with a fork and is opaque all the way through.

● Italian Style Flounder
(Phases II and III)

2 pounds flounder fillets

1/2 tablespoon organic unsalted butter

Salt and pepper to taste

1 tablespoon lemon juice

1/2 cup fresh tomato, diced

2 teaspoons dried basil

1 teaspoon garlic powder

Directions

1. Preheat oven to 350°.

2. Arrange flounder in a medium-sized baking dish. Dot with butter, season with salt and pepper, and sprinkle with lemon juice. Top with tomato, basil, and garlic powder.

3. Cover, and bake 30 minutes in the preheated oven, or until fish is easily flaked with a fork.

● Fish & Eggplant in Curry Tomato Sauce (Phases II and III)

1 can (14.5 oz.) tomatoes, diced or crushed

1 tablespoon olive oil

3 cloves of garlic

1/2 small onion (optional)

1 tablespoon curry powder

1 tablespoon caraway seeds (optional)

3/4 teaspoon oregano

3/4 teaspoon thyme

Salt and cayenne pepper to taste (optional)

1-1/2 pound of white fish fillet (sole, flounder, turbot)

2 medium or large eggplants, peeled and cut into medium size chunks

1/2 cup fresh cilantro or parsley for garnish, chopped

Directions

1. Prepare the sauce in a large Pyrex bowl and mix all ingredients except for the cilantro, parsley, and eggplant.

2. Clean and wash the fish fillet with filtered or spring water.

3. Marinate the fish in the Pyrex bowl with the sauce.

4. Preheat oven to 375° and cook the fish in the sauce for one hour.

5. Place the eggplant chunks in a steamer and cook until they are soft (about 15 minutes).

6. Remove fish from oven, add the steamed eggplant and mash it all together with a fork. Garnish with chopped, fresh cilantro or parsley.

You'll be surprised how large this dish looks; however, it's very light and delicious. Fish meals go very well with steamed carrots, broccoli, cauliflower, rice, millet, and corn.

● Baked Red Snapper
(Phases II and III)

1 medium whole red snapper

2 large onions, sliced

3 ripe tomatoes, sliced

5 lemons

4 cloves of garlic, fine chopped

3 tablespoons olive oil

Salt and pepper to taste

Directions

1. Preheat oven to 375°.

2. Clean the fish of all scales.

3. Place 1/3 of the onion and tomato slices on the bottom of a baking pan. Sprinkle a portion of the garlic on the onion and tomatoes. Squeeze the juice of one lemon onto them.

4. Rub fish with salt and pepper, and place on the onions and tomatoes.

5. Stuff 1/3 of the onion, tomato, and garlic inside the belly of the snapper. Place the remaining 1/3 onion, tomato, and garlic on top of the snapper.

6. Cut one lemon into slices and place around top of fish. Squeeze juice of the remaining lemon over top of the fish. Drizzle olive oil over the fish.

7. Cover fish with aluminum foil. Cook for 40–50 minutes, depending on the size of the fish. To test for doneness: poke fish with a fork—the meat should be flaky.

Chapter 14

Questions and Answers

Q: Can I take estrogen inhibitors with other supplements?

A: Estrogen-inhibiting supplements can be safely taken with other supplements. Estrogen inhibitors (flavones and indoles), as listed in Chapter 5, are derived from botanical sources that have shown to be both safe and beneficial in helping treat ailments.

These extracts do not adversely interfere with vitamins, minerals, or antioxidants. In fact, it is highly recommended to take them with a multivitamin supplement to maximize the benefits of both supplements in lowering the metabolic stress on the body.

Q: My problem is stubborn belly fat. I've tried virtually every fat-loss program with no results. What makes the Anti-Estrogenic Diet different?

A: Most fat-loss programs today have failed to even address the problem of excess estrogen nor do they offer any solution for stubborn fat. Conversely, the Anti-Estrogenic Diet was designed to specifically address estrogen-related disorders including stubborn fat. The foods incorporated in the diet and estrogen-inhibiting supplements have demonstrated the capacity to exert anti-estrogenic effects. This helps create a metabolic environment that favors the breakdown of estrogen-sensitive fatty tissues, including areas that generally resist fat-burning.

Q: Should I take isoflavone supplements for treating estrogen-related disorders?

A: Products made with isoflavones (mostly from soy) often claim to help balance estrogen, help alleviate symptoms related to estrogen disorders, and even lower the risk for cancer. Products in this category are targeted mostly toward women. The theory behind this group of products is that isoflavones can bind to estrogen receptors and by occupying them, prevent estradiol (a most potent estrogen hormone) from binding and acting. According to this theory, being estrogen mimickers, isoflavones would induce a mild estrogenic effect while blocking estradiol from inducing its highly potent estrogenic effect.

There are studies that indeed support this theory. Unfortunately, there is also growing evidence that, under certain conditions, estrogen mimickers may do just the opposite. Certain isoflavones, including those derived from soy and black cohosh, were found to induce an estrogenic effect that may actually accelerate the problem (of an existing estrogen disorder) by increasing an already elevated level of excess estrogen in the body. Some studies indicate that isoflavones are part of the problem, not the solution.

Unlike estrogen mimickers, the estrogen inhibitors listed in Chapter 5 have no estrogenic ingredients, nor do they have any inherent estrogenic activity. In conclusion, to be on the safe side, do not apply estrogen-promoting substances to treat disorders related to excess estrogen.

Q: What is the difference between the estrogen inhibitors that you list in the book and steroid inhibitors in addressing estrogen-related fat gain?

A: Some fat-loss products are made with so-called "suicidal" steroid inhibitors. Products in this category are targeted mostly toward men. The theory behind these products is that they contain certain steroidal substances that can bind to the aromatase enzyme, responsible for synthesizing estrogen from androgens. The inhibition of this enzyme could in theory help lower estrogen levels in men, thus helping them to lose fat. The problem with this theory is that it overlooks the high probability of side effects. Virtually all steroidal substances come with the price of side effects. Notable among them are estrogen kickbacks, which are also associated with delayed fat-gain rebounds and a decline in testosterone levels.

Unlike steroid inhibitors, the estrogen inhibitors we recommend for the diet have no inherent steroidal activity. They are a combination of plant-based estrogen inhibitors that exclusively provide a triple-action effect in lowering excess estrogen. Furthermore, they inhibit estrogen via different mechanisms than steroid inhibitors and cause no side effects such as estrogen kickbacks or fat-gain rebound. Distinctively different from steroid inhibitors, they come with a clear dietary guideline. When incorporated as part of the Anti-Estrogenic Diet, they may help eliminate stubborn fat and sustain a lean, healthy body in the long run.

Q: I am under estrogen-replacement therapy. Could an estrogen-inhibitor supplement counteract my HRT?

A: The estrogen inhibitors listed in the book will not counteract your HRT. If anything, they will help defend your body from increased levels of harmful estrogen metabolites often associated with the use of estrogen drugs. Thus, when incorporated together with the Anti-Estrogenic Diet, they may help lower the health risk involved with HRT.

Q: How long will it take before I actually begin to lose weight?

A: You should already be able to notice weight loss from the jump-start phases. Virtually all those on the Anti-Estrogenic Diet have experienced weight loss by the end of the first week (Phase I). Nonetheless, it generally takes about 2–3 weeks for the estrogen inhibitors extracts to reach a peak loading state in the body with the maximum anti-estrogenic effect. If your weight gain is estrogen-related, you may need to apply the diet and supplements for 2–3 weeks before reaching an optimum on-going, slimming-down effect in stubborn fat areas.

Q: Is coffee helpful in losing weight?

A: When used properly, naturally caffeinated beverages such as coffee or tea can actually be more beneficial than for just losing weight. Both coffee and tea have shown to possess neural protective and anti-cancerous properties. When freshly brewed or processed, coffee and tea contain flavones and phenols that help protect the body from tissue damage and aging. Both coffee and tea can help enhance cognitive functions with a sense of controlled alertness. Both caffeinated beverages are mild adrenal stimulators and thus promote energy expenditure and fat burning. Nevertheless, both are regarded as recreational drugs and, if abused, could cause addiction and adrenal fatigue.

For that matter, restrict the serving size and frequency of caffeinated beverages to the bare minimum needed for a pick-me-up. In the case of coffee, try not to exceed more than two cups per day. Another alternative is to have a smaller serving such as a half shot of espresso instead of a double espresso. Use your common sense and instincts. Do not habitually overload yourself with coffee as a solution for chronic sleep deprivation. Energy crushes and cravings for sweets or coffee could be related to a lack of sleep. Try to treat the core of your problem. If you suffer from an existing health condition such as hypertension, consult with your physician before having any caffeinated beverages or stimulants.

In conclusion, coffee and tea can be helpful in enhancing weight loss. Just be careful as to how much and how often you consume them.

Q: I am physically lean and fit. Should I supplement my diet with estrogen inhibitors and practice the Anti-Estrogenic Diet for maintenance?

A: It is virtually impossible to completely avoid estrogenic chemicals in the environment, food, and water. Regardless of your fitness level, you should protect your body from the harmful effects of xenoestrogens. For that matter, estrogen-inhibitor extracts should be incorporated together with anti-estrogenic food as a means to sustain a viable nutritional defense against the ever-growing onslaught of chemicals in today's world.

Q: I am over 40 and already suffer from a declining testosterone level and a low libido. Can the Anti-Estrogenic Diet help boost my vigor?

A: There is growing evidence that estrogenic chemicals accelerate aging, which is also associated with a decline in testosterone. The Anti-Estrogenic Diet may help counteract this process by providing the body with both anti-estrogenic and testosterone-boosting nutrients. If you take supplemental DHEA, you may also be able to minimize its conversion to estrogen and thereby induce maximum androgenic effect. To boost your libido, train your body to shift from carb to fat fuel. Try to increase the intake of food listed in Phase II of the diet. Raw nuts and seeds, when eaten with the right combination of foods and in large amounts, could be the best fuel for improving your libido.

Q: Is the Anti-Estrogenic Diet geared more toward women than men?

A: The diet is for both men and women. Nonetheless, due to higher levels of circulating estrogen in women than in men, the Anti-Estrogenic Diet often affects women more quickly than it does men. Men, however, may instantly benefit from its anti-estrogenic hormonal balancing and protective effects. The Anti-Estrogenic Diet may help boost libido, performance, and also help increase men's capacity to become leaner, as well as develop a higher resilience to disease.

Q: I suffer from Type II diabetes. In spite of taking prescription drugs, my blood sugar is chronically elevated. The doctor offers me no solution besides increasing the dosage of drugs. What should I do to treat my condition?

A: Type II diabetes is a condition that can be naturally reversed. We have already addressed diabetes and blood sugar problems in previous chapters of the book. Nevertheless, let me note again how important it is to avoid all moderate and high glycemic foods, including all grains, potatoes, yams, fruits, and all sugars until your blood sugar stabilizes below 100 for at least six weeks. It would most likely take about that period of time for the body to reset its glucose tolerance and insulin sensitivity. Meanwhile, incorporate legumes, nuts, and seeds as your main fuel foods. Maintain the right food combinations. Supplement your diet with all essential nutrients as well as estrogen inhibitors. That way, you'll be able to gradually lower the metabolic stress on the liver and thus improve its capacity to utilize glucose. As glucose utilization improves, the liver will be able to regain its capacity to regulate blood lipids. That will consequently lead to the lowering of both blood sugar and blood lipids. Ultimately, this will lead to the reversal of your condition.

Q: Will I lose muscle mass during the jump-start of the diet?

A: If you follow the guidelines in the book, you will not lose muscle mass. In fact, it is very likely that you may even gain. The jump-start phases will help increase your body's capacity to utilize nutrients, including amino acids in the muscle tissues. The incorporation of liver-detoxifying and hormone-boosting nutrients can help enhance recuperation and promote an anabolic potential in the body. Even though protein selection is quite limited in the initial phases, one can still take advantage of post-exercise recovery meals and nourish the muscles with sufficient amounts of amino acids for recuperation and growth. The book provides detailed guidelines for physically active individuals that may be applied at any phase of the diet.

Q: Is the Anti-Estrogenic Diet based on the same principles as the Warrior Diet?

A: Yes and no. Both diets are based on survival principles. Both diets provide clear guidelines on human eating cycles and food priorities. Both diet programs promote detox, fuel utilization, and sustained energy. Both are also effective in weight loss. Nonetheless, while the Warrior Diet revolutionizes the old concepts of nutrition and exercise, the Anti-Estrogenic Diet breaks new ground in guiding individuals about how to protect against excess estrogen. Unlike the Warrior Diet, the Anti-Estrogenic Diet provides alternative plans to those who wish to keep a traditional routine of eating breakfast, lunch, and dinner. In other words, the Anti-Estrogenic Diet applies Warrior Diet principles in a way that is geared more toward mainstream, average lifestyles. Excess estrogen is a global ecological problem that affects all people today—men, women, and children alike. The Anti-Estrogenic Diet program was therefore designed to provide practical solutions for everyone of any age, gender, ethnic group, or culture.

Q: Are progesterone creams based on wild yams effective in promoting progesterone?

A: Progesterone creams and herbal products containing wild yam extract are being sold under the guise that they carry bioactive ingredients that will convert into progesterone and DHEA in the body, and thereby help balance estrogen and give relief of estrogen-disorder symptoms.

Unfortunately, all human studies indicate that claims for wild yam-based creams and products may be bogus. The active ingredient in wild yam—diosgenin—was found to possess no progesterone bioactivity nor does it elevate progesterone or DHEA levels in humans.

Q: Is licorice estrogenic? Is it safe?

A: Licorice is definitely estrogenic. It may also cause water retention. Licorice contains active isoflavones; notable among them is glabrene that has shown various degrees of estrogen-receptor-promoting activities. Recent studies showed that licorice's isoflavones, glabrene and isoliquiritigenin, can bind to human estrogen receptors with high affinity, and affect the body's tissues in a manner similar to estradiol.

Furthermore, the glycyrihitinic acid, found in licorice, contributes to the aldosterone-like actions of licorice—aldosterone being a mineral-corticosteroid hormone that causes water retention in the body. Note that deglycerinized licorice (DGL) also retains high estrogen-receptor-binding activity.

In conclusion, all kinds of licorice are estrogenic and should be avoided in cases of disorders associated with excess estrogen.

Q: Can progesterone-receptor-binding isoflavones help promote progesterone?

A: Virtually all progesterone-binding isoflavones were found to be either neutral or progesterone antagonists. That includes isoflavones from various herbs, including red clover and licorice, that have shown high levels of PR-binding with progesterone-suppressing effects. For that matter, herbs such as red clover and licorice are estrogenic and progesterone suppressive. To be on the safe side, avoid progesterone-inhibiting herbs in cases of disorders associated with excess estrogen and declining progesterone.

Q: Can I have beer once in a while?

A: You can have beer once in a while, but watch out for how much and how often you consume it. Even though beer contains less alcohol than wine or other alcoholic beverages, it may cause more estrogenic effects than any other plain alcoholic drinks. There are two reasons for this.

First, typical beer consumption per sitting is much higher than consumption of wine or other beverages. Just look at the super gigantic size of a beer mug, compared to wine or vodka glasses. Second, beer has significant amounts of phytoestrogens from hops—a bitter-herb ingredient in beer—which is highly estrogenic. Based on recent studies, researchers at the University of California concluded that hops contain ER-binding phytoestrogens, thereby supporting previous anecdotal evidence of the estrogen-promoting effect of this herb. The double-wham effect of beer can be overwhelming. High alcohol intake combined with highly estrogenic substances can devastate the body with a strong estrogenic effect, often leading to an increase in size of estrogen-sensitive fatty tissues in the belly, leading to the so-called "beer belly."

In conclusion, if you like to have a beer once in a while, have a glass of beer instead of a mug. Do not binge drink. If you suffer from an existing estrogen-related disorder or stubborn belly fat, avoid drinking beer until you notice a substantial improvement in your condition.

A Final Note

According to Newton's third law of thermodynamics, life is a constant struggle against the universal forces of entropy. Without the means to resist these forces of degradation, any living organism would lose its ability to sustain its integral structure, and consequently cease to exist. Each living thing, including we humans, carries survival mechanisms that when triggered, induce metabolic actions that protect the body against destructive forces, which cause disorders, disease, and death.

Food provides us with the fuel for our survival machine. Anything that threatens the integrity of our nutrition is detrimental to our life. For that matter, estrogenic substances that have penetrated our food and water supply are destroying our lifelines, rendering them toxic and virtually unsuitable for human or animal consumption.

The Anti-Estrogenic Diet was created to address this specific problem and also provide solutions. Please consult our website for free useful information including more recipes, food preparation methods, scientific references, as well as nutritional supportive services, testimonials, supplements, and other advice you may need to sustain and enjoy the Anti-Estrogenic Diet.

● ● ● **To learn more, log on to www.DefenseNutrition.com or call 1-866-927-3438.**

Appendix:
Estrogen Inhibitors—Science Overview

What really promotes estrogen and what doesn't? The purpose of this addendum is to provide a scientific overview of some of the most important and controversial estrogen inhibitors.

Flavonoids

It has been widely established that certain compounds in plants called flavonoids can exert various biological effects, including antioxidant, anti-carcinogenic, and anti-estrogenic as well as other modulation of sex hormones. Flavonoids are a group of polyphenolic phytochemicals including flavones, isoflavones, isoflavonones, catechins and chalcones, among other chemicals. They occur in relatively high concentration in fruits, vegetables, nuts, and grains. Flavonoids are known to have widely diverse and beneficial biological effects, such as anti-inflammatory (Middelton, 1998), antioxidant (Pletta, 2000), anti-viral (Jassim and Naji, 2003), and anti-cancerous (Alercreutz, 2002; Frei and Higdon, 2003; Rietveld and Wiseman, 2003). They also modulate the function of sex hormones and their receptors.

Estrogen promoters vs. estrogen inhibitors

Certain flavonoids, such as the isoflavone genistein (found in soy), are estrogenic (Wang et al., 1996; Zand et al., 2000); whereas others, such as 5.7 dihydroxyflavone (chrysin), are anti-estrogenic and can interfere with steroid hormone synthesis and metabolism.

Note that estrogen-promoting compounds are often called phytoestrogens. However, only a limited number are in fact estrogen receptor agonists (estrogen mimickers). In contrast, many flavonoids are known to interfere, to a greater or lesser degree, with various cytochrome P 450 enzymes, including those involved in steroid hormone synthesis.

Several studies have addressed the ability of flavonoids to interfere with the activity or expression of aromatase (cytochrome P 450 19 cyp19), the enzyme responsible for the conversion of androgens to estrogens (Ibrahim and Abul-Hajj, 1990; Kellis and Vickery, 1984; Le Ball et al., 1998; Whitehead and Lacey, 2003). These studies revealed significant differences in the relative inhibition potencies of flavonoids. For that matter, cellular uptake and metabolism capacity of flavonoids as well as their tissue-specific affinity need to be considered.

Aromatase inhibition of flavonoids

The ability of various natural flavonoids to inhibit aromatase activity was investigated and documented. For example, quercitine (abundant in onion and garlic) was found to inhibit human aromatase activity in placental microsomes (Kellis and Vickery, 1984). The ranking of relative inhibition potencies differed among tissue tests, although some general trends are apparent. In certain cancerous cells (placental chorlocarcinoma cells), apigenine (derived from chamomile) was more potent than hydroxyflavone, chrysin (derived from passiflora), naringenin (derived from grapefruit), and quercitine. On the other hand, in normal human placental cells, 7 hydroxyflavone and chrysin were more potent than apigenine, naringenin, and quercitine. In general, studies show that flavones (chrysin, apigenine) were more potent aromatase inhibitors than flavonones (7 hydroxyflavone or naringenin), a finding that is consistent with previous reports (Le Bail et al., 1998; Sorrinen et al., 2001).

Researchers have found no effect of 7 methoxyflavone and flavonone on aromatase inhibition. For that matter, products containing methoxylated flavones that were previously introduced to the fitness industry failed to provide any substantial estrogen inhibitory benefits.

Aromatase induction by flavonoids

The human aromatase enzyme is known to be under the control of several tissue-specific promoters (Bulun et al., 2003; Harodo et al., 1993; Simpson et al., 1993). For example, aromatase in human gonads is regulated through promoter P 11 and 1.3, both of which are stimulated by cAMP-dependent protein kinase A (PKA) second messenger pathway. Healthy breast adipose stromal tissue utilizes promoter 1.4, which is stimulated by the glucocorticoid (cortisol) signaling pathway. However, in malignant breast tumors, a promoter switch appears to occur, resulting in strongly increased activity levels of promoters P 11 and 1.3 (Agrawald et al., 1996; Kamatetal, 2002). Researchers believe that the above promoters are therefore important in aromatase regulation in gonads and breast tumors.

Dutch researchers have found that certain flavones that cause fat loss in animal studies may induce aromatase activity in humans. For instance, the isoflavone genistein has been shown to increase intracellular cAMP concentrations and thus cause elevation of cAMP-mediated P 11 and 1.3 promoter-specific mRNA levels. The researchers indicated that aromatase-inducing isoflavones are known to be phosphodiestrase inhibitors in several tissues. Phosphodiestrase is the enzyme that metabolizes cAMP, thus lowering its cellular level. Inhibition of phosphodiesterase will sustain high levels of cAMP, a cellular factor that induces fat breakdown in adipose tissue. Both quercitin and genistein have been shown to stimulate cAMP-mediated Lipolysis in rat adipocytes (Kuppusamy and Das, 1992). However, they also have been shown to induce aromatase activity in cancer cells. Quercitine, however, was found to be an aromatase inhibitor in healthy cells or when applied to cancer cells in high concentration.

Note that forskolin (derived from coleus as forskolii), a compound used by the fitness industry to promote fat loss, should be consumed with caution, if at all. Forskolin is a potent estrogen promoter due to its cAMP-stimulating and aromatase-inducing effects. Researchers have been using forskolin as a standard aromatase-promoting agent for comparative purposes.

Balancing estrogen promoters with estrogen inhibitors

Because the average human diet contains several flavonoids with aromatase-inhibitory properties in various concentrations, scientists speculate that it is possible for combined tissue concentrations to be reached via proper supplementation, and thus result in a certain degree of aromatase inhibition.

Nonetheless, under normal dietary conditions, flavones occur in complex mixtures, with often-contradictory effects (inhibiting as well as promoting) on the aromatase enzyme and estrogen metabolism. Therefore it has been suggested that consumption of high concentrations of potent aromatase-inhibiting compounds (more than 100 times the typical diet) may result in high concentrations of single flavonoids, sufficient to inhibit aromatase activity.

Inhibition of aromatase activity in individuals suffering from over-estrogenic activity due to exposure to chemicals, use of hormonal therapy, or adverse effects of aging may help reduce the risk for cancer and may also help eliminate estrogen-related fat gain.

Recent studies at the Medical University of South Carolina, Charleston, led researchers to the conclusion that flavones work better when combined together to provide total body (systemic) aromatase inhibition and defense against estrogen. Flavones such as chrysin, apigenine, and galangin (an ingredient in bee propolis) showed various inhibition and different affinities (potencies) toward the two human cytochrome P 450 aromatase enzymes: 1A1 and 1A2. Therefore, combining anti-aromatase flavones will most likely grant a superior total body estrogen-inhibiting impact by virtue of addressing various tissue-specific ratios of CYP 1A1 / CUP 1A2.

Biochemical mechanisms of aromatase-inhibition potencies of flavonoids

It has been established that the most important contributor to the aromatase-inhibitory effect of flavonoids is the 4-oxo group on the c-ring of the flavone base structure (Kao et al., 1998). Hydroxylation of the 7-position on the A-ring enhances the inhibitory potency considerably (such as with 7 hydroxy flavone and chrysin-5, 7 dihydroxyflavone). Scientists did not observe a dramatic difference in potency when comparing 7 hydroxy flavone with 5, 7 dihydroxyflavone. As noted, it has also been established that flavonones such as naringenin (from grapefruit) have lower aromatase-inhibitory potency than flavones. It is plausible that the lack of 2, 3 double-bond in the flavonones results in reduced electro-negativity of the 4-oxo group and subsequently, a weaker interaction of this group with the heme prosthetic group of the aromatase enzyme.

The mechanism by which isoflavones such as those found in soy fail to exhibit aromatase-inhibition capacity is attributed to the fact that when flavonoid structures are substituted on the 3 position of the c-ring, as was observed for genistein, there is a consequent obliteration of aromatase-inhibition capacity. This is consistent with the very weak or non-existent inhibitory effects of these compounds found in studies (Campbell and Kruzer, 1993; Kao et al., 1998; Polissero et al., 1996; Saarinen et al., 2001).

Aromatase-inhibiting potency values of natural flavonoids

In a recent review—*Toxicological Sciences 82,* pp. 70–79 (2004)—researchers at Utrecht University, Netherlands, and the University of California, Davis, published a comparative database of aromatase-inhibiting potencies by natural flavonoids.

Various classes of naturally occurring flavonoids including flavons, flavonones, isoflavones, and catechins were tested for their effects on aromatase activity and cell viability in human adrenocortical carcinoma cells.

Among the flavones, 7 hydroxyflavone, chrysin, and to a lesser degree apigenine have shown aromatase-inhibiting activities in concentrations of about 4, 7 and 20 µM, respectively (micron µM – 0.001 milliliter), values well below concentrations that caused the first sign of cutotoxicity. The first statistical signs of significant decreases in cell viability of about 20% were observed at 30 µM for chrysin, and at 100 µM for 7-oh flavone and apigenine. 7 methoxyflavone had no statistically significant effect on aromatase activity at concentrations up to 100 µM, a concentration at which the first statistically significant decrease in cell viability of about 30% was observed.

The flavonones were considerably less potent aromatase inhibitors than the flavones: 7-hydroxyflavonone and naringenine had aromatase-inhibiting potencies close to the high concentrations of 100 µM, a level at which both compounds cause a 20% decrease in a cell's viability. 7 methoxyflavonone had no effect on aromatase activity but nonetheless caused a 15% decrease in cell viability at a cellular concentration of 100 µM.

Finally, the flavonoids catechins and epicatechins (found in green tea) have shown no aromatase-inhibiting potencies. Both flavonoids have shown no cellular toxicity effects.

CLA

A certain compound in dairy has been shown to possess anti-estrogenic and anti-carcinogenic properties. Called CLA (conjugated linoleic acid), this compound is an ingredient in milk fat, with higher levels found in milk derived from grass-fed cows. CLA is also found in human mothers' milk. Statistically, high levels of CLA in breast milk have been correlated with decreased cancer incidence in both mothers and their offspring. Australian researchers found that consumption of CLA significantly reduced circulating LDL cholesterol in humans. CLA was found to inhibit a certain protein (called apolipoprotein B 100), responsible for the production of LDL cholesterol in the liver.

Studies at Bassett Research Institute, Cooperstown, New York, revealed that CLA decreased tumor growth in animals. Other studies at the University of Alberta, Edmonton, Canada, have shown that CLA can destroy cancer cells in humans. Both CLA and omega-3 oil (N-3) were found to interfere with tumor cell cycles and induce apoptosis (cell suicide) in cancer cells.

Scientists believe that CLA works via similar mechanisms as N-3. Substantial evidence supports the claims for anti-estrogenic/anti-carcinogenic properties of CLA. Recent studies at the University of Texas, Department of Medicine/Clinical Immunology indicated that CLA directly inhibits the growth of human breast cancer cells. CLA selectively inhibited proliferation of estrogen receptor positive (ER+) breast cancer cells.

Studies at Emory University, in Atlanta, Georgia, provided evidence that the anti-estrogenic activity of CLA is caused by inactivating estrogen receptors. Previous studies showed that CLA can inhibit estrogen-related transcriptional activity in the genes, and thereby induce an anti-tumor effect on breast cancer cells.

CLA constitutes a group of conjugated fatty acid isomers with a variety of biological effects. One notable effect is the reduction of body fat in animals. It has been suggested that the active isomers regarding weight loss are the trans-10, cis-12 (t10c12) and the cis-9, trans-11 (c9t11). Studies in humans, however, indicated that even though CLA might slightly decrease body fat, particularly belly fat, there is no evidence that CLA affects body mass index or body weight in humans. Moreover, scientists at the University of Uppsala, Sweden, found that the same CLA isomer that induces fat reduction in animals unexpectedly caused insulin resistance in humans. The evidence isn't yet conclusive, and more studies are needed to investigate the effect of CLA on insulin sensitivity. Interestingly, researchers at Friedrich Schiller University of Jena, Germany, found that the same CLA isomer that has been suspected of causing insulin resistance—CLA cis-9, trans-11 (c9t11) isomer, also called rumenic acid—inhibits the growth of leukemia cells.

In conclusion, studies have shown that CLA isomers demonstrate profound anti-estrogenic and anti-cancerous effects. However, CLA failed to induce substantial fat loss in humans and it may also adversely affect insulin sensitivity. New studies are required to examine isomer-specific effects of CLA in animals and humans.

Flaxseed's Lignans

There is substantial evidence that flaxseed and its lignans (components in the fiber) inhibit estradiol carcinogenic effects.

Researchers at the Division of Oncology, Faculty of Health Sciences, University Hospital, Linkoping, Sweden, found that certain phytoestrogens in flaxseeds (enterodiol and enterolactone) counteracted the effects of estradiol (E2) and thereby inhibited the growth and angiogenesis (growth of blood vessels) in solid tumors in mice. Both flaxseed phytoestrogens (lignan-derived) decreased the secretion of VEGF—vascular endothelial growth factor—in human breast cancer cells.

The researchers concluded that flaxseed and its lignans have potent anti-estrogenic effects on estrogen receptors and may be beneficial in breast cancer prevention.

Note: One of the main sources of phytoestrogens in the Western diet is lignans. Plant lignans such as those found in flaxseeds and sesame seeds appear in their naturally occurring state in the form of a compound called SDG (secoisolariciresinol diglucoside). SDG is metabolized by gut bacteria (microflora) to the more bioactive mammalian lignans enterodiol and enterolactone.

Sesame's Lignans

Sesame ingestion has been shown to improve blood lipids in humans and provide antioxidative effects in animals. Sesamin, a sesame lignan, was recently reported to be converted by intestinal microflora to enterolactone, the same phytoestrogen (metabolite) that has been derived from flaxseed lignans. Studies at the Department of Human Development and Family Studies, National Taiwan Normal University, Taipei, have shown that sesame ingestion benefited post-menopausal women by improving blood lipids, antioxidant status, and possibly sex hormone status. Most notable was the dramatic increase (72%) in urinary 2 hydroxyestrone, which is the highly beneficial "anti-estrogenic" metabolite of estrogen. High levels of 2 hydroxyestrogens have been correlated with a lower risk for estrogen-related cancer in women and men. For that matter, sesame phytoestrogens were found to provide beneficial anti-estrogenic effects similar to those resulting from ingestion of cruciferous indoles (in broccoli, cauliflower, and cabbage) by shifting estrogen metabolism to favor the production of beneficial "anti-estrogenic" metabolites, rather than harmful estrogen metabolites.

Glossary

agonist: A chemical, drug, or substance that can combine with a receptor on a cell to promote a physiological reaction.

antagonist: A substance that can bind with a receptor on a cell to inhibit a physiological reaction.

androgen: A male sex hormone, produced in the testes and adrenals, that is responsible for typical male sexual characteristics.

anti-estrogenic: A term used to describe a substance that suppresses, inhibits, or counterbalances estrogen activity when introduced into the body.

antioxidant: A substance or nutrient that counteracts and neutralizes oxygen free radicals, which are toxins and byproducts of body metabolism and energy production.

anti-inflammatory: A substance or nutrient that counteracts the inflammatory process. These include anti-oxidants, omega-3 oils, and protease enzymes.

aromatase: An enzyme or group of enzymes that promotes the conversion of an androgen (such as testosterone) into estrogen.

conjugated linoleic acid (CLA): A group of fatty-acid isomer compounds found in milk fat, which have shown anti-estrogenic and anti-cancerous properties, but may decrease insulin sensitivity.

co-factor: A substance that acts with another substance to bring about certain physiological effects.

cruciferous vegetables: Broccoli, cauliflower, brussels sprouts, and other cabbage-family edible plants. These contain highly bioactive, estrogen-modulating indoles.

endogenous: Occurring within the body.

Hormone Replacement Therapy (HRT): Usually denotes a therapy for women using the estrogen hormone (or estrogen combined with progesterone) to help alleviate the adverse effects of menopause.

estrogen receptor (ER): A molecular structure or site on the outside or inside of a cell, particularly sensitive to and able to bind with estrogen.

estrogen: A natural steroidal hormone secreted by the ovaries, placenta, adipose (fat) tissue, and testes that stimulates the development of female secondary sex characteristics, and promotes the growth and maintenance of the female reproductive system.

estrogen inhibitors: Substances that can help decrease, hinder, or inhibit estrogen activity in the body. Also have the capacity to interfere with estrogen metabolism and shift it to favor the production of beneficial metabolites.

estrogenic: A characteristic of certain chemicals or substances that can mimic or promote estrogen activity in the body.

estrogenic chemicals: Industrial chemicals having a structure and action similar to estrogen. They are found in the natural and man-made environment in numerous products, plastics, food, and water.

estrogen dominance: A condition where there is an excess of estrogen in the body over other hormones such as progesterone (in women) or testosterone (in men).

excess estrogen: See **estrogen dominance**

isoflavone: A type of phytoestrogen found in legumes, grains, spices, and herbs; the highest levels are found in soy.

lipids: Fatty compounds.

liver: An organ responsible for regulating critical metabolic functions including the regulation of lipid and glucose metabolism and the neutralization and detoxification of steroidal hormones, chemical substances, and waste toxins.

liver detoxification : A process that involves removal of toxins from the liver.

menopause: The gradual cessation of a woman's menstrual cycle. Usually occurs between the ages of 40 and 50.

organic: A term used to describe a nutritional product or food that is cultivated, produced, and processed without the use of chemicals, pesticides, hormones, or harmful additives.

perimenopause: A phase of a woman's life before the onset of menopause, often marked by a various physical signs such as hot flashes and menstrual irregularity. Also known as premenopause.

phenotype: An observable, physical trait of an organism based on genetic and environmental influences.

phytoestrogen: A naturally occurring estrogenic compound found in plants; has a capacity to bind to estrogen receptors and either promote or inhibit estrogen in the body.

probiotics: "Friendly" gut bacteria that counteract the actions of pathogenic bacteria in the digestive tract. Also helps detoxify and metabolize byproducts of digestion.

progesterone: A steroidal hormone, predominantly in women, that has an estrogen-balancing effect. Is secreted by the ovaries and the adrenal glands. Acts to prepare the uterus for implantation of the fertilized ovum, to maintain pregnancy, and to promote development of the mammary glands.

progesterone receptors (PR): A molecular structure or site on the outside or inside of a cell that is particularly sensitive to and able to bind with progesterone.

Syndrome X: A term used to describe a condition in which obesity, blood sugar problems, elevated blood lipids, and high blood pressure are present, all of which are often associated with elevated levels of circulating estrogen.

testosterone: A male steroidal hormone, produced by the testes, that stimulates the development of male sex organs, secondary sexual characteristics, and sperm. Testosterone counterbalances estrogen activity.

xenoestrogens: See **estrogenic chemicals**

References

Adlecreutz, H. 1998. Human health and phytoestrogens. In *Reproductive and Developmental Toxicology,* Ed. K. S. Korach. New York: Marcel Dekker, 299–371.

Adlercreutz, H. 2002. Phyto-oestrogens and cancer. *Lancet Oncol* 3:364–373.

Agarwal, V. R., S. E. Bulun, M. Leitch, R. Rohrich, and E. R. Simpson. 1996. Use of alternative promoters to express the aromatase cytochrome P450 (CYP19) gene in breast adipose tissues of cancer-free and breast cancer patients. *J Clin Endocrinol Metab* 81:3843–3849.

Agatha, G., A. Voigt, E. Kauf, and F. Zintl. 2004. Conjugated linoleic acid modulation of cell membrane in leukemia cells. *Cancer Lett* 209 (1):87–103.

Albertazzi P., F. Pansini, G. Bonaccorsi, L. Zanotti, D. Forini, and D. de Aloysio. 1998. The effect of soy supplementation on hot flashes. *Obstet Gynecol* 91:6–11.

Allred, C. D., K. F. Allred, Y. H. Ju, S. M. Virant, and W. G. Helferich. 2001. Soy diets containing varying amounts of genistein stimulate growth of estrogen-dependent (MCF-7) tumors in a dose-dependent manner. *Cancer Res* 61:5045–5050.

Aminot-Gilchrist, D. V., and H. D. Anderson. 2004. Insulin resistance-associated cardiovascular disease: potential benefits of conjugated linoleic acid. *Am J Clin Nutr* 79 (5 Suppl):1159S–1163S.

Anderson, D., M. M. Dobrzynska, and N. Basaran. 1997. Effect of various genotoxins and reproductive toxins in human lymphocytes and sperm in the comet assay. *Teratog Carcinog Mutagen* 17:29–43.

Arai, Y., S. Watanabe, M. Kimira, K. Shimoi, R. Mochizuki, and N. Kinae. 2000. Dietary intakes of flavonols, flavones, and isoflavones by Japanese women and the inverse correlation between quercetin intake and plasma LDL cholesterol concentration. *J Nutr* 130:2243–2250.

Barret, J. 2005. Phthalates and Baby Boys: Potential Disruption of Human Genital Development. *Environ Health Perspect* Aug. 113 (8): A542).

Bennetts, H. W., E. J., Underwood and F. L. Shier. 1946. A breeding problem of sheep in the south-west division of Western Australia. *J Dept Agric West Aust* 23:142.

Blake, C.A., Ashiru, O.A. 1997. Disruption of rat estrous cyclicity by the environmental estrogen 4-tert-octylphenol. *Proc Soc Exp Biol Med* 216:446-451.

Bravo, L. 1998. Polyphenols: chemistry, dietary sources, metabolism, and nutritional significance. *Nutr Rev* 56:317–333.

Brueggemeier, R.W., Bhat, A.S., Lovely, C.J., Coughenour, H.D., Joomprabutra, S., Weitzel, D.H., Vandre, D.D., Yusuf, F., Burak, W.E. 2001. 2-Methoxymethylestradiol: a new 2-methoxy estrogen analogue that exhibits antiproliferation activity and alters tubulin dynamics. *J Steroid Biochem Mol Biol* 78:145-156.

Bulun, S. E., S. Sebastian, K. Takayama, T. Suzuki, H. Sasano, and M. Shozu. 2003. The human CYP19 (uromatase P450) gene: update on physiologic roles and genomic organization of promoters. *J Steroid Biochem Mol Biol* 86:219–224.

Campbell, D. R., and M. S. Kurzer. 1993. Flavonoid inhibition of aromatase enzyme activity in human preadipocytes. *J Steroid Biochem Mol Biol* 46:381–388.

Carreau, S., S. Lambard, C. Delalande, I. Denis-Galeraud, B. Bilinska, and S. Bourguiba. 2003. Aromatase expression and role of estrogens in male gonad: a review. *Reprod Biol Endrocrinol* 1:35.

References

Cassidy, A. 1996. Physiological effects of phyto-oestrogens in relation to cancer and other human health risks. *Proc Nutr Soc* 55:399–417.

Center for Food Safety and Applied Nutrition. 1993. *Priority-based assessment of food additives (PAFA) database.* Washington, DC: US Food and Drug Administration, 58.

Chorazy, P. A., S. Himelhoch, N. J. Hopwood, N. G. Greger, and D. C. Postellon. 1995. Persistent hypothyroidism in an infant receiving a soy formula: case report and review of the literature. *Pediatrics* 96:148–150.

Colborn, T., Dumanoski, D., Myers, J.P. 1996. Our stolen future: Are we threatening our fertility, intelligence, and survival? *A Scientific Detective Story.* Plume, New York.

Collomb, M., R. Sieber, and U. Butikofer. 2004. CLA isomers in milk fat from cows fed diets with high levels of unsaturated fatty acids. *Lipids* 39 (4):355–64.

Colon, I., Caro, D., Bourdony, C.J., Rosario, O. 2000. Identification of phthalate esters in the serum of young Puerto Rican girls with premature breast development. *Environ Health Perspect* 108: 895-900.

Constantinou, A., K. Kiguchi, and E. Huberman. 1990. Induction of differentiation and strand breakage in human HL-60 and K-562 leukemia cells by genistein. *Cancer Res* 50:2618–2624.

Cotroneo, M. S., and C. A. Lamartiniere. 2001. Pharmacologic, but not dietary, genistein supports endometriosis in a rat model. *J Toxicol Sci* 61:68–75.

Crisp, T.M., Clegg, E.D., Cooper, R.L., Wood, W.P., Anderson, D.G., Baetcke, K.P., Hoffmann, J.L., Morrow, M.S., Rodier, D.J., Schaeffer, J.E., Touart, L.W., Zeeman, M.G., Patel, Y.M. 1998. Environmental endocrine disruption: An effects assessment and analysis. *Environ Health Perspect* 106:11-56.

Dauchy, R. T., E. M. Dauchy, L. A. Sauer, D. E. Blask, L. K. Davidson, J. A. Krause, and D. T. Lynch. 2004. Differential inhibition of fatty acid transport in tissue–isolated steroid receptor negative human breast cancer xenografts perfused in situ with isomers of conjugated linoleic acid. *Cancer Lett* 209 (1):7–15.

Daxenberger, A., Ibarreta, D., Meyer, H. 2001. Possible health impact of animal oestrogens in food. *Human Reprod Update* 7(3): 340-355.

de Veth, M. J., J. M. Griinari, A. M. Pfeiffer, and D. E. Bauman. 2004. Effect of CLA on milk fat synthesis in dairy cows: comparison of inhibition by methyl esters and tree fatty acids, and relationships among studies. *Lipids* 39 (4):365–72.

Divi, R. L., H. C. Chang, and D. R. Doerge. 1997. Anti-thyroid isoflavones from soybean isolation, characterization, and mechanisms of action. *Biochem Pharmacol* 54:1087–1096.

Duncan, A. M. 1999. Hormonal effects of soy isoflavone in pre- and post-menopausal women. Dissertation, University of Minnesota.

Durgam, V. R., and G. Fernandes. 1997. The growth inhibitory effect of conjugated linoleic acid on MCF-7 cells is related to estrogen response system. *Cancer Lett* 116 (2):121–30.

Erlund, I., M. L. Silaste, G. Alfthan, M. Rantala, Y. A. Kesaniemi, and A. Aro. 2002. Plasma concentrations of the flavonoids hesperetin, naringenin and quercetin in human subjects following their habitual diets, and diets high or low in fruit and vegetables. *Eru J Clin Nutr* 56:891–898.

Eyjolfson, V., L. L. Spriet, and D. J. Dyck. 2004. Conjugated linoleic acid improves insulin sensitivity in young, sedentary humans. *Med Sci Sports Exerc* 36 (5):814–20.

Field, C. J, and P. D. Schley. 2004. Evidence for potential mechanisms for the effect of conjugated linoleic acid on tumor metabolism and immune function: lessons from n-3 fatty acids. *Am J Clin Nutr* 79 (6 Suppl):1190S–1199S.

Frei, B., and J. V. Higdon. 2003. Antioxidant activity of tea polyphenols in vivo: evidence from animal studies. *J Nutr* 133:3275S–3284S.

Gaullier, J. M., J. Halse, K. Hoye, K. Kristiansen, H. Fagertun, H. Vik, and O. Gudmundsen. 2004. Conjugated linoleic acid supplementation for 1 y reduces body fat mass in healthy overweight humans. *Am J Clin Nutr* 79 (6):1118–25.

Guo, Y.L., Hsu, P.C., Hsu, C.C., Lambert, G.H. 2000. Semen quality after prenatal exposure to polychlorinated biphenyls and dibenzofurans. *Lancet* 356:1240-1241.

Harada, N., T. Utsumi, and Y. Takagi. 1993. Tissue-specific expression of the human aromatase cytochrome P-450 gene by alternative use of multiple exons 1 and promoters, and switching of tissue-specific exons 1 in carcinogenesis. *Proc Nat Acad Sci USA* 90:11312–11316.

Hargreaves, D. F., C. S. Potten, C. Harding, et al. 1999. Two-week dietary soy supplementation has an estrogenic effect on normal premenopausal breast. *J Clin Endocrinol Metab* 84:4017–4024.

Harris, C.A., Henttu, P., Parker, M.G., Sumpter, J.P. 1997. The estrogenic activity of phthalate esters in vitro. *Environ Health Perspect* 105:802-811.

Harrison, P.T., Holmes, P., Humfrey, C.D. 1997. Reproductive health in humans and wildlife: Are adverse trends associated with environmental chemical exposure? *Sci Total Environ* 205:97-106.

Hashimoto, Y., Moriguchi, Y., Oshima, H., Nishikawa, J., Nishihara, T., Nakamura, M. 2000. Estrogenic activity of chemicals for dental and similar use in vitro. *J Mater Sci Mater Med* 11:465-468.

Hendrich, S., G. J. Wang, H. K. Lin, et al. 1999. *Isoflavone metabolism and bioavailability. In: Antioxidant Status, Diet, Nutrition and Health,* ed. A. M. Papas. Boca Raton: CRC Press, 221–230.

Howdeshell, K., Hotchkiss, A.K., Thayer, K.A., Vandenbergh, J.G., vom Saal, F.S. 1999. Exposure to bisphenol A advances puberty. *Nature* 401:762-764.

Hydovitz, J. D. 1960. Occurrence of goiter in an infant on a soy diet. *N Engl J Med* 262:351–3.

Ibrahim, A. R., and Y. J. Abul-Haij. 1990. Aromatase inhibition by flavonoids. *J Steroid Biochem Mol Biol* 37:257–260.

Jassim, S. A., and M. A. Naji. 2003. Novel antiviral agents: a medicinal plant perspective. *J Appl Microbiol* 95:412–427.

Ju, Y. H., C. D. Allred, K. F. Allred, K. L. Karko, D. R. Doerge, and W. G. Helferich. 2001. Physiological concentrations of dietary genistein dose-dependently stimulate growth of estrogen-dependent human breast cancer (MCF-7) tumors implanted in athymic nude mice. *J Nutr* 131:2957–2962.

Jungeström, M.B., L.U. Thompson, and C. Dabrosin. 2007. Flaxseed and its lignans inhibit estradiol-induced growth, angiogenesis, and secretion of vascular endothelial growth factor in human breast cancer xenografts in vivo. *Clin Cancer Res* 13: 1061-1067.

Kaiser, J. 2000. Hazards of particles, PCBs focus of Philadelphia meeting. *Science* 288:424-425.

Kamat, A., M. M. Hinshelwood, B. A. Murry, and C. R. Mendelson. 2002. Mechanisms in tissue-specific regulation of estrogen biosynthesis in humans. *Trends Endocrinol Metab* 13:122–128.

Kao, Y. C., C. Zhou, M. Sherman, C. A. Laughton, and S. Chen. 1998. Molecular basis of the inhibition of human aromatase (estrogen synthetase) by flavone and isoflavone phytoestrogens: A site-directed mutagenesis study. *Environ Health Perspect* 10685–92.

Kellela, K., K. Heinonen, and H. Saloniemi. 1984. Plant oestrogens: the cause of decreased fertility in cows. A case report. *Nordisk Veterinaermedicin* 36:124–129.

Kellis, J. T., Jr., and L. E. Vickery. 1984. Inhibition of human estrogen synthetase (aromatase) by flavones. *Science* 225:1032–1034.

Kelly, G. E., C. Nelson, M. A. Waring, G. E. Joannou, and A. Y. Reeder. 1996. Metabolites of dietary (soya) isoflavones in human urine. *Clin Chim Acta* 223:9–22.

Knight, D. C., and J. A. Eden. 1994. A review of the clinical effects of phytoestrogens. *Obstet Gynecol* 87:897–904.

Kulling, S. E., and M. Metzier. 1997. Induction of micronuclei, DNA strand breaks and HPRT mutations in cultured Chinese hamster V79 cells by the phytoestrogens coumoestrol. *Food Chem Toxicol* 35:605–613.

Kuntz, S., U. Wenzel, and H. Daniel. 1999. Comparative analysis of the effects of flavonoids on proliferation, cytotoxicity, and apoptosis in human colon cancer cell lines. *Eur J Nutr* 38:133–142.

Kuppusamy, U. R., and N. P. Das, 1992. Effects of flavonoids on cyclic AMP phosphodiesterase and lipid mobilization in rat adipocytes. *Biochem Pharmacol* 44:1307–1315.

Le Bail, J. C., Y. Champavier, A. J. Chulia, and G. Habrioux,. 2000. Effects of phytoestrogens on aromatase, 3beta and 17beta-hydroxysteroid dehydrogenase activities and humanbreast cancer cells. *Life Sci* 66:1281–1291.

Le Bail, J. C., T. Laroche, F. Marre-Founier, and G. Habrioux. 1998. Aromatase and 17beta-hydroxysteroid dehydrogenase inhibition by flavonoids. *Cancer Lett* 133: 101–106.

Leopold, A. S., M. Erwin, J. Oh, and B. Browning. 1976. Phytoestrogens: adverse effects on reproduction in California quail. *Science* 191:98–100.

Liu, J., and N. Sidell. 2005. Anti-estrogenic effects of conjugated linoleic acid through modulation of estrogen receptor phosphorylation. *Breast Cancer Res Treat* 94 (2):161–9.

Manach, C., A. Scalbert, C. Morand, C. Remesy, and L. Jimenez. 2004. Polyphenols: food sources and bioavailability. *Am J Clin Nutr* 79:727–747.

Mattson, M. 2005. The need for controlled studies of the effects of meal frequency on health.

Lancet 365:1978-80.

McLachlan, J.A., Newbold, R.R., Bullock, B.C. 1980. Long-term effects on the female mouse genital tract associated with prenatal exposure to diethylstilbestrol. *Cancer Res* 40:3988-3999.

McMichael-Phillips, D. F., C. Harding, and M. Morton, et al. 1998 Effects of soy-protein supplementation on epithelial proliferation in histologically normal human breast. *Am J Clin Nutr* 68:1431S–1436S.

Middleton, E., Jr. 1998. Effect of plant flavonoids on immune and inflammatory cell function. *Adv Exp Med Biol* 439:175–182.

Moore, N.P. 2000. The oestrogenic potential of the phthalate esters. *Reprod Toxicol* 14:183-192.

Moral, R., Russo, J., Balogh, G.A., Mailo, D.A., Russo, I.H., Lamartiniere, C. 2005. Compounds in plastic packaging acts as environmental estrogens altering breast genes. *96th Annual Meeting of the American Association for Cancer Research.*

Munro, I. C., M. Harwood, J. J. Hlywka, A. M. Stephen, J. Doull, W. G. Flamm, and H. Adlercreutz. 2003. Soy isoflavones: a safety review. *Nutr Rev* 61 (1):1–33.

Nadal, A., Ropero, A.B., Laribi, O., Maillet, M., Fuentes, E., Soria, B. 2000. Nongenomic actions of estrogens and xenoestrogens by binding at a plasma membrane receptor unrelated to estrogen receptor a and estrogen receptor b. *Center for Scientific Studies of Santiago.*

Nagata, C., S. Inaba, N. Kawakami, T. Kakizoe, and H. Shimizu. 2000. Inverse association of soy product intake with serum androgen and estrogen concentrations in Japanese men. *Nutr Cancer* 36:14–18.

References

Newbold, R. R., E. P. Banks., B. Bullock, W. N. Jefferson. 2001. Uterine adenocarcinoma in mice treated neonatally with genistein. *Cancer Res* 61:4325–4328.

Oh, Y. S., H. S. Lee, H. J. Cho, S. G. Lee, K. C. Jung, and J. H. Park. 2003. Conjugated linoleic acid inhibits DNA synthesis and induces apoptosis in TSU-Prl human bladder cancer cells. *Anticancer Res* 23 (6C):4765–72.

Ohno, S., S. Shinoda, S. Toyoshima, H. Nakazawa, T. Makino, and S. Nakajin. 2002. Effects of flavonoid phytochemicals on cortisol production and on activities of steroidogenic enzymes in human adrenocortical H295R cells. *J Steroid Biochem Mol Biol* 80:355–363.

O'Shea, M., J. Bassaganya-Riera, and I. C. Mohede. 2004. Immunomodulatory properties of conjugated linoleic acid. *Am J Clin Nutr* 79 (6 Suppl):1199S–1206S.

Pelissero, C., M. J. Lenczowski, D. Chinzi, B. Davail-Cuisset, J. P. Sumpter, and A. Fostier. 1996. Effects of flavonoids on aromatase activity, an in vitro study. *J Steroid Biochem Mol Biol* 57:215–223.

Petrakis, N. L., S. Barnes, E. B. King, et al. 1996. Stimulatory influence of soy protein isolate on breast secretion in pre- and postmenopausal women. *Cancer Eipdemiol Biomarkers Prev* 5:785–794.

Price, K. R., and G. R. Fenwick. 1985. Naturally occurring oestrogens in food. A review. *Food Addit Contam* 2:73–106

Quella, S. K., C. L. Leprinzi, and D. L. Barton, et al. 2000. Evaluation of soy phytoestrogens for the treatment of hot flashes in breast cancer survivors: a north central cancer treatment group trial. *J Clin Oncol* 18:1068–1074.

Rainer, L., and C. J. Heiss. 2004. Conjugated linoleic acid: health implications and effects on body composition. *J Am Diet Assoc* 104 (6):963–8.

Rao, C. V., C-X. Wang, and B. Simi, et al. 1997. Enhancement of experimental colon cancer by genistein. *Cancer Res* 57:3717–3722.

Recchia, A.G., Vivacqua, A., Gabriele, S., Carpino, A., Fasanella, G., Rago, V., Bonofiglio, D., Maggiolini, M. 2004. Xenoestrogens and the induction of proliferative effects in breast cancer cells via direct activation of oestrogen receptor alpha. *Food Additives & Contaminants* 21:134-144.

Riserus, U., B. Vessby, J. Arnlov, and S. Basu. 2004. Effects of cis-9, trans-11 conjugated linoleic acid supplementation on insulin sensitivity, lipid peroxidation, and proinflammatory markers in obese men. *Am J Clin Nutr* 80 (2):279–03.

Routhledge, E.J., White, R., Parker, M.G., Sumpter, J.P. 2000. Differential effects of xenoestrogens on coactivator recruitment by estrogen receptor (ER) alpha and ERb. *J Biol Chem* 46:35986-35993.

Saarinen, N., S. C. Joshi, M. Ahotupa, X. Li, J. Ammala, S. Makela, and R. Santti. 2001. No evidence for the in vivo activity of aromatase-inhibiting flavonoids. *J Steroid Biochem Mol Biol* 78:231–239.

Safe, S. 2000. Endocrine disruptors and human health—is there a problem? An update. *Environ Health Perspect* 108:487-493.

Sanderson, J. T., J. Boerma, G. W. Lansbergen, and M. van den Berg. (2002). Induction and inhibition of aromatase (CYP19) activity by various classes of pesticides in H295R human adrenocortical carcinoma cells. *Toxicol Appl Pharmacol* 182:44–54.

Sanderson, J. T., J. Hordijk, M. S. Denison, M. F. Springsteel, M. H. Nantz, and M. van den Ber. 2004. Induction and inhibition of aromatase (CYP10) activity by natural and synthetic flavonoids compounds in H295R human adrenocortical carcinoma cells. *Toxicol Sci* 82:70–79.

Sanderson, J. T., W. Seinen, J. P. Giesy, and M. van den Berg. 2000. 2-Chloro-s-triazine herbicides induce aromatase (CYP19) activity in H295R human adrenocortical carcinoma cells: a novel mechanism for estrogenicity? *Toxicol Sci* 54:121–127.

References

Santell, R. C., Y. C. Chang, M. G. Nair, and W. G. Helferich. 1997. Dietary genistein exerts estrogenic effects upon the uterus, mammary gland and the hypothalamic/pituitary axis in rats. *J Nutr* 127:263–269.

Setchell, K. D. R., S. J. Gosselin, and M. B. Welsh, et al. 1987. Dietary estrogens: a probable cause of infertility and liver disease in captive cheetahs. *Gastroenterology* 93:225–233.

Shafie, S., Brooks, S. 1977. Effect of prolactin on growth and the estrogen receptor level of breast cancer cells (MCF-7). *Cancer Res* 37:792-799.

Shepard, T. H., and G. E. Pyne, J. F. Kirschvink, M. McLean. 1960. Soybean goiter. *N Engl J Med* 262:1099–1103.

Simpson, E. R., M. S. Mahendroo, G. D. Means, M. W. Kilgore, C. J. Corbin, and C. R. Mendelson. 1993. Tissue-specific promoters regulate aromatase cytochrome P450 expression. *Clin Chem* 39:317–324.

Singleton, D.W., Feng, Y., Chen, Y., Busch, S.J., Lee, A.V., Puga, A., Khan, S.A. 2004. Bisphenol-A and estradiol exert novel gene regulation in human MCF-7 derived breast cancer cells. *Mol Cell Endocrinol* 221:47-55.

Singleton, D.W., Feng, Y., Yang, J., Puga, A., Lee, A.V., Khan, S.A. 2005. Gene expression profiling reveals novel regulation by bisphenol-A in estrogen receptor-alpha-positive human cells. *Environ Res Online* Nov. 2005.

Sohoni, P., Sumpter, J.P. 1998. Several environmental oestrogens are also anti-androgens. *J Endocrinol* 158:327-339.

Song, T. T., S. Hendrich, and P. A. Murphy. 1999 Estrogenic activity of glycitein, a soy isoflavone. *J Agric Food Chem* 47:1607–1610.

Sower, S.A., Reed, K.L>, Babbitt, K.J. (2000). Limb malformations and abnormal sex hormone concentrations in frogs. *Environ Health Perspect* 108:1085-1090.

Tanmahasamut, P., J. Liu, L. B. Hendry, and N. Sidell. 2004. Conjugated linoleic acid blocks estrogen signaling in human breast cancer cells. *J Nutr* 134 (3):674–80.

Teede, H. J., F. S. Dalais, D. Kotsopoulos, Y-L. Liang, S. Davis, and B. P. McGrath. 2001. Dietary soy has both beneficial and potentially adverse cardiovascular effects: a placebo-controlled study in men and post-menopausal women. *J Clin Endocrinol Metab* 86:3053–3060.

Terpstra, A. N. 2004. Effect of conjugated linoleic acid-on body composition and plasma lipids in humans; an overview of the literature. *Am J Clin Nutr* 79 (3):352–61.

Thain, R. I. 1965. Bovine infertility possibly caused by subterranean clover: a preliminary report. *Aust Vet J* 41:277–281.

Thylor, C. G., P. Zahradka. 2004. Dietary conjugated linoleic acid and insulin sensitivity and resistance in rodent models. *Am J Clin Nutr* 79:11645–11685.

Turner, R. T., B. L. Riggs, and T. C. Spelsberg. 1994. Skeletal effects of estrogen. *Endocrinol Rev* 15:275–300.

Van Wyk, J. J., M. B. Arnold, J. Wynn, and F. Pepper. 1959. The effects of a soybean product on thyroid function in humans. *Pediatrics* 24:752–760.

Wada, H., Tarumi, H., Imazato, S., Narimatsu, M., Ebisu, S. 2004. In vitro estrogenicity of resin composites. *J Dent Res* 83:222-226.

Walsh, D.E., Dockery, P., Doolan, C.M. 2005. Estrogen receptor independent rapid non-genomic effects of environmental estrogens on [CA^{++})i in human breast cancer cells. *Mol Cell Endocrinol* 230:23-30.

Wang, T. T., N. Sathyamoorthy, and J. M. Phang. 1996. Molecular effects of genistein on estrogen receptor mediated pathways. *Carcinogenesis* 17:271–275.

References

Wang, Y. W., and P. J. Jones. 2004. Conjugated linoleic acid and obesity control: efficacy and mechanisms. *Int J Obes Relat Metab Disord* 28 (8):941–55.

Wang, Y., and P. J. Jones. 2004. Dietary conjugated linoleic acid and body composition. *Am J Clin Nutr* 79 (6 Suppl):1153S–1158S.

Wantanabe, M. and S. Nakajin. 2004. Forskolin up-regulates aromatase (CYP19) activity and gene transcripts in the human adrenocortical carcinoma cell line H295R. *J Endocrinol* 180: 125–133.

White, L., H. Petrovitch, G. W. Ross, and K. Masaki. 1996. Association of mid-life consumption of tofu with late life cognitive impairment and dementia: The Honolulu-Asia aging study. *Neurobiol Aging* 17:S121.

White, L., H. Petrovitch, and F. W. Ross, et al. 1996. Prevalence of dementia in older Japanese-American men in Hawaii: The Honolulu-Asia aging study. *JAMA* 276:955–960.

White, L., H. Petrovitch, and G. W. Ross, et al. 2000. Brain aging and midlife tofu consumption. *J Am Coll Nutr* 19:242–255.

Wilcox, A.J., Baird, D.D., Weinberg, C.R., Hornsby, P.O., Herbst, A.L. 1995. Fertility in men exposed prenatally to diethylstilbestrol. *N Engl J Med* 332:1411-1416.

Willingham, E., Rhen, T., Sakata, J.T., Crews, D. 2000. Embryonic treatment with xenobiotics disrupts steroid hormone profiles in hatchling red-eared slider turtles (Trachemys scripta elegans). *Environ Health Perspect* 108:329-332.

Wiseman, H. 1997. Dietary phytoestrogens: disease prevention versus potential hazards. *Nutr Food Sci* 1:32–38.

Wozniak, A.L., Nataliya, N.B., Watson, C.S. 2005. Xenoestrogens at picomolar to nanomolar concentrations trigger membrane estrogen receptor-a-mediated $Ca?^+$ fluxes and prolactin release in GH3/B6 pituitary tumor cells. *Environ Health Perspect* 113(4): 431-439.

Wu, W., Y. Kang, N. Wang, H. Jou, and T. Wang. 2006. Sesame ingestion affects sex hormones, antioxidant status, and blood lipids in postmenopausal women. *J Nutr* 36: 1270-1275.

Zand, R. S., Jenkins, D.J., and Diamandis, E.P. 2000. Steroid hormone activity of flavonoids and related compounds. *Breast Cancer Res Treat* 62:35–49.

Zava, D. T., C. M. Dollbaum, and M. Blen. 1998. *Estrogen and progestin bioactivity of foods, herbs and spices* (44247). *Proc Soc Exper Biol Med* 217 (3):369–78.

Zhai, S., R. Dai, F. K. Friedman, and R. E. Vestal. 1998. Comparative Inhibition of Human Cytochromes P450 1A1 and 1A2 by Flavonoids. *Drug Metab Disposition* 26 (10):989–992).

Zhan, W., Xu, Y., Li, A.H., Zhang, J., Schramm, K.W., Kettrup, A. 2000. Endocrine disruption by hexachlorobenzene in Crucian Carp (Carassius auratus gibelio). *Bull Environ Contam Toxicol* 65:560-566.

Zhang, J. G., M. A. Tirmenstein, F. A. Nicholls-Grzemski, and M. W. Fariss. 2001. Mitochondrial electron transport inhibitors cause lipid peroxidation-dependent and-independent cell death: protective role of antioxidants. *Arch Biochem Biophys* 393:87–96.

Zheng, W., Q. Dai, and L. J. Custer, et al. 1999. Urinary excretion of isoflavonoids and the risk of breast cancer. *Cancer Epidemiol Biomarkers Prev* 8:35–40.

Zhou, X., C. Sun, L. Jiang, and H. Wang. 2004. Effect of conjugated linoleic acid on PPAR gamma gene expression and serum leptin in obese rat. *Wei Sheng Yan Jiu* 33 (3): 307–9.

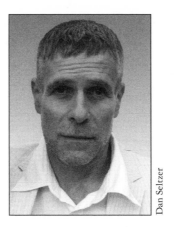

Dan Seltzer

About the Author

ORI HOFMEKLER is a modern renaissance man whose life has been driven by two passions: art and health. His formative experience as a young man with the Israeli Special Forces prompted a life interest in diet and fitness regimes that help improve human survival.

After the army, Hofmekler attended the Bezalel Academy of Art and the Hebrew University, Jerusalem, where he studied art, philosophy, and biology, and received a degree in Human Sciences. A world-renowned painter best known for his controversial political satire, Hofmekler's work has been featured in magazines and newspapers worldwide, including *Time, Newsweek, L'Express, Die Zeit, Der Spiegel, New York Times, People, Rolling Stones, Esquire, The New Republic,* and *Playboy,* as well as *Penthouse,* where he was a monthly columnist for seventeen years and health editor from 1998–2000.

Hofmekler has published two books of political art: *Hofmekler's People* and *Hofmekler's Gallery.* As founder, editor-in-chief, and publisher of *Mind and Muscle Power,* a national health and fitness magazine, he introduced his Warrior Diet to the public in a monthly column to immediate acclaim from readers and professionals in the health and fitness fields.

Having numerous readers worldwide, *The Warrior Diet* has been translated into Italian and French, and featured in health and lifestyle magazines as well as the prestigious medical journal *The Lancet.*

Hofmekler's dietary and training methods have been endorsed by nutritional and medical experts, scientists, champion athletes and martial artists, and military and law enforcement instructors, as well as by authors of best-selling books.

The Warrior Diet, LLC and Defense Nutrition, LLC currently provide nutrition and training workshops for their followers, as well as certification seminars for health experts, medical clinicians, coaches, trainers, and military and law enforcement instructors. Hofmekler resides with his wife and children in Woodland Hills, California.

RICK OSBORN, co-editor of *The Anti-Estrogenic Diet,* has a long-time love for and interest in the areas of health, nutrition, and fitness. He first met Ori Hofmekler through the Warrior Diet program and is currently marketing and projects director at Defense Nutrition, LLC. Osborn lives in Raleigh, North Carolina.

● ● ● **Contact us at www.DefenseNutrition.com or call us at: 1-866-927-3438**

Index

Index